Art Therapy with Special Education Students

Art Therapy with Special Education Students is a practical and innovative book that details the best suitable ways to work in the field of art therapy with special education students.

This book provides the reader with practical approaches, techniques, models, and methodologies in art therapy that focus on special education students, such as those with autistic spectrum disorder, attention deficit hyperactivity disorder, learning disabilities, behavioral disorders, and students with visual and hearing impairments. Each chapter addresses a specific population, including an overview of the literature in the field, along with descriptions of practices derived from interviews with experienced art therapists who specialize in each population. The chapters cover the therapeutic goals of each population, the specific challenges, intervention techniques, and the meaning of art. Dedicated working models that have emerged in the field and collaborative interventions involving parents and staff members, along with clinical illustrations, are also available throughout the book.

Art therapists and mental health professionals in the school system will appreciate this comprehensive collection of contemporary work in the field of art therapy with special education students.

Dafna Regev is an art therapist and researcher. She is an associate professor, head of the art therapy program, and member of the Emili Sagol Creative Arts Therapies Research Center at the University of Haifa, Israel.

DAFNA REGEV

Art Therapy with Special Education Students

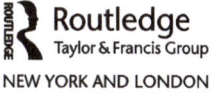
Routledge
Taylor & Francis Group

NEW YORK AND LONDON

Cover image: Getty Image

First published 2023
by Routledge
605 Third Avenue, New York, NY 10158

and by Routledge
4 Park Square, Milton Park, Abingdon, Oxon, OX14 4RN

Routledge is an imprint of the Taylor & Francis Group, an informa business

© 2023 Dafna Regev

The right of Dafna Regev to be identified as author of this work has been asserted in accordance with sections 77 and 78 of the Copyright, Designs and Patents Act 1988.

Library of Congress Cataloging-in-Publication Data
A catalog record for this title has been requested

ISBN: 978-0-367-74282-9 (hbk)
ISBN: 978-0-367-74281-2 (pbk)
ISBN: 978-1-003-15691-8 (ebk)

DOI: 10.4324/9781003156918

Typeset in Joanna MT
by codeMantra

Contents

Contents

Preface

For many years I have been intrigued by the interrelationships between art therapy and the education system. It was clear to me that there was tremendous potential for observing students as whole individuals, and that amazing work is being done by the art therapists working in this field. However, my years of work as an art therapist in the education system left me with the feeling that a variety of difficulties and burdens sometimes makes it difficult to realize this potential. My bachelor's degree is in special education and psychology, so these two branches of special education and therapy have been ingrained in me since the beginning of my academic career. My M.A. and Ph.D. focused on art therapy, but were done in the Department of Education at the University of Haifa. I have continued to move between the two fields by coordinating a number of special education tracks. Today, I head the art therapy program at the University of Haifa, which was founded a little over a decade ago.

Over the past few years, my research has increasingly focused on arts therapy in the education system. I conduct research jointly with Prof. Sharon Snir from Tel Hai College and in full cooperation with the national supervisors of arts therapies at the Special Education Division of the Israel Ministry of Education. This collaboration has led us over the years to explore the views and issues facing arts therapists who work in the education system.

We began publishing our studies in 2015 to map out the advantages and disadvantages of integrating art therapy into the education system. We interviewed 131 people from the education system including art therapists, supervisors, educators, counselors, and principals working in the Jewish and Arab educational systems. We primarily discovered the complexity of this fabric, and how much investment is required by all involved before students and families can really be given quality art therapy that also resonates with the remainder of the time students spent in the education system (Belity et al., 2016; Keinan et al., 2016; Regev et al., 2015; Snir et al., 2017). A later study conducted completed the exploration of the clients' perspectives when we interviewed adolescents about their perceptions of art therapy in the education system (Harpazi et al., 2020). We were thrilled to see that there are students whose prime reason for going to school is art therapy, where the art therapists are sometimes referred to as "Mom", which shows their importance to them.

Subsequently, we began to delve more deeply into the therapeutic process of art therapy in the education system. We wondered what it looked like from the art therapists' point of view and asked them to document the course of their work, their deliberations and questions, goals, interventions, and ways of working in diary form (Adoni-Kroyanker et al., 2018). The analysis pointed to the need to think more deeply about the therapeutic approaches used by art therapists with clients in the education system, given the frequent need to work with short-term models. Other art therapists were asked to document the most helpful and hindering events in their sessions in art therapy (Shakarov et al., 2019). We found that both the therapeutic relationship between the art therapist and the client or group, and the observation of the artworks were perceived by the therapists as promoting their therapeutic work. In addition, we asked ourselves about the nature of relationships between process variables (e.g., the therapeutic alliance, client involvement in therapy, etc.) and outcome variables in these therapies (Keidar et al., 2021; Regev, 2022). The findings provided a complex picture that showed that it is important to continue to delve into this issue.

The next step was to observe the art therapy room in the education system (Danieli et al., 2019; Dornai et al., 2019). This led to the formulation of a more grounded statement about what art therapists consider to be important in their art therapy rooms. In an exploratory study, we found that there was a correlation between the art therapists' more positive perceptions of the location of the room, the suitability of its equipment, the art materials and furnishings, and improvement in outcome measures. By probing their working conditions, we also examined the relationship with their job satisfaction and burnout (Elkayam et al., 2020). The findings pointed to the importance of teamwork and the extent to which it is related to satisfaction in art therapists. In addition, we found that the more they were satisfied with the working conditions in the art therapy room assigned to them in the education system, the less they reported exhaustion.

In recent years, we have examined much more specific issues often voiced by art therapists working in the education system. For example, we investigated parent–child art psychotherapy in the education system, which has begun to develop in response to the acknowledgment of the value of working in parallel with students' parents (Tamir & Regev, 2020). We also responded to calls from national supervisors in the special education division of the education system to examine issues related to maternity leave, how to deal with suspended treatment, and the national obligation to fill these hours (Raubach Kaspi et al., 2022).

In 2021, we published a book on arts therapies in the education system. This volume, which was also published by Routledge (Taylor and Francis), represents the voice of arts therapists who have worked for years in the education system and have found creative ways of adapting their work to the system (Regev & Snir, 2021). Interacting with these arts therapists revealed the importance of the dissemination of knowledge in the field. It underscored that our job as researchers is primarily to gather data and to give this information meaning and conceptualization. Working on this book was not easy, but it moved me on a personal level and made it clear that contact in the field is extremely valuable. I emerged with a need to understand the ways in which art therapists work with a variety of special education populations. Two events in my life contributed to the writing of this volume. The first is that I went on sabbatical and writing is something I really enjoy doing. The second impetus derived from my teaching an "Art Therapy with Children and Youth" course, in which I sometimes felt that my knowledge of these specific populations needed to be updated, and that the best source of this information could come from the art therapists who work with these students in the education system on a daily basis.

When I first planned the book, I did not imagine what the year would look like. It was the year of COVID, and I found myself in my art therapy room reading about working with students in the education system and mostly interviewing dozens of art therapists who were struggling to give these students the best therapy possible in unprecedented conditions. The conversations with these art therapists took on enormous meaning but most of all emphasized how much thought, creativity, depth, and sometimes even courage are mustered by these art therapists. The book you have in your hands today would not have been possible without the contribution of each and every one of them, and I thank them from the bottom of my heart.

This volume is composed of eight chapters, which outline different ways of working in art therapy with the main populations of students in the Israeli education system. The first chapter deals with art therapy with students with learning disabilities (LD) and attention-deficit/hyperactivity disorder (ADD/ADHD). These students are most often integrated within the regular education system, where they are seen by art therapists who help them deal with the emotional and social issues that are sometimes associated with these difficulties. The second and third chapters cover art therapy with students with sensory impairments. The second chapter focuses on students who are deaf or hard of hearing (D/HH), while the third concentrates on blind students or those with a Severe Visual Impairment (B/SVI). These students sometimes continue to study in the regular education system or attend frameworks designed for students in special education, depending on their condition and degree of functioning. When they are integrated into the regular system, art therapists need to find ways to tailor their work to them. The fourth chapter discusses art therapy with students on the autism spectrum disorder (ASD). These students also study in a variety of settings in the education system depending on their level of functioning. This chapter addresses the specific challenges of students at different levels of functioning, and how these different levels require different types of interventions.

The fifth and sixth chapters are devoted to art therapy with students in special education settings. The fifth chapter deals with students with intellectual and developmental disabilities (IDD), and the sixth chapter presents approaches to students with Behavioral Disorders. The challenges of working with these students vary considerably. The art therapists shared their ways of working and the difficulties they face in countertransference. Finally, the last two chapters have to do with art therapy for students in hospitals. In the State of Israel, the education system employs art therapists in the framework of schools located in hospitals. The seventh chapter explores hospitalized students who are coping with a variety of illnesses that require hospitalization for varying lengths of time. The eighth and final chapter deals with students with mental disorders. These students can be found on the entire spectrum from hospitalization in closed or open psychiatric wards to in day hospitalization settings where students are treated until they can be re-integrated into the community in special education schools. Most often, these students go back and forth between these frameworks.

I hope that reading this book will shed new light on the goals, challenges, and interventions in art therapy with each of these populations. Each chapter discusses the similarities and differences in approaches of the art therapists interviewed here. The chapters deal with the therapeutic power of art with these students as well as the specific ways in which art therapists enable parents and staff to connect and communicate with them. At the end of each chapter, a case illustration is presented. Importantly, these examples do not depict actual cases but rather combine observations and insights from the work of the therapists I interviewed. They provide a composite of the nature of case work related to the specific populations described in each chapter.

One of the personal outcomes of working on this book was my heightened interest in making videos of the art therapists in their art therapy rooms in the education system, as they show and explain how they work. With the approval of the Ethics Committee of the Ministry of Education and the support of the Emili Sagol Creative Arts Therapies Research Center at the University of Haifa, this project has begun. The films can be found at https://catrc.haifa.ac.il/index.php/research-projects-4/project. I hope that in the near future we will also be able to provide subtitles in English, for those interested outside of Israel.

REFERENCES

Adoni-Kroyanker, M., Regev, D., Snir, S., Orkibi, H., & Shakarov, I. (2018). Practices and challenges in implementing art therapy in the school system. *International Journal of Art Therapy*, 24(1), 40–49.

Belity, I., Regev, D., & Snir, S. (2016). Supervisors' perceptions of art therapy in the Israeli education system. *International Journal of Art Therapy*, 22(3), 96-105.

Danieli, Y., Snir, S., Regev, D., & Adoni- Kroyanker, M. (2019). Suitability of the art therapy room and changes in outcome measures in the education system. *International Journal of Art Therapy*, 24(2), 68–75.

Dornai, H., Snir, S., & Regev, D. (2019). Therapy rooms for art therapy in the Israeli educational system. *The Academic Journal of Creative Arts Therapies*, 9(2) 887–900 (In Hebrew).

Elkayam, C., Snir, S., & Regev, D. (2020). Relationships between work conditions, job satisfaction and burnout in Israeli Ministry of Education art therapists. *International Journal of Art Therapy*, 25(1), 35–38.

Harpazi, S., Regev, D., Snir, S., & Raubach Kaspi, R. (2020). Perceptions of art therapy in adolescent clients treated within the school system. *Frontiers in Psychology*, 11, 3025.

Keidar, L., Snir, S., Regev, D., Orkibi, H., & Adoni-Kroyanker, M. (2021). Relationship between the therapist-client bond and outcomes of art therapy in the Israeli school system. *Art Therapy*, 38(4), 189–196.

Keinan, V., Snir, S., & Regev, D. (2016). Art therapy in the Israeli educational system – Teachers' perspectives. Canadian Art Therapy Association Journal, 29(2), 67–76.

Raubach Kaspi, R., Snir, S., Regev, D., & Harpazi, S. (2022). Art therapists', supervisors' and school counselors' perceptions of the substitute art therapist's role in the education system during maternity leave. *International Journal of Art Therapy*, 27(1), 26–35.

Regev, D. (2022). A process-outcome study in school-based art therapy. *International Journal of Art Therapy*, 27(1), 17–25.

Regev, D., Green-Orlovich, A., & Snir, S. (2015). Art therapy in schools – The therapist's perspective. *The Arts in Psychotherapy*, 45, 47–55.

Regev, D., & Snir, S. (Eds.). (2021). *Integrating art therapy into education: A collective volume*. Routledge (Taylor & Francis Group).

Shakarov, I., Regev, D., Snir, S., Orkibi, H., & Adoni- Kroyanker, M. (2019). Helpful and hindering events in art therapy as perceived by art therapists in the educational system. *The Arts in Psychotherapy*, 63, 31–39.

Snir, S., Regev, D., Alkara, M., Belity, I., Green-Orlovich, A., Daoud, H., Melzak, D., Mekel, D., Salamey, A., Abd Elkader, H., & Keinan, V. (2017). Art therapy in the Israeli education system – A qualitative meta-analysis. *International Journal of Art Therapy*, 23(4), 169–179.

Tamir, R., & Regev, D. (2020). Characteristics of parent-child art psychotherapy in the education system. *The Arts in Psychotherapy*, 72, 101725.

Acknowledgments

First and foremost, I would like to thank Anat Marnin-Shaham, the national supervisor of arts therapies at the Special Education Division of the Israel Ministry of Education, who is always so willing to help me. This time as well, Anat enabled me to compile the list of interviewees for the book and engage in discussions as to which populations would be the most important to present. Second, I would like to thank all the art therapists who participated in this book, from the bottom of my heart. They opened their doors to me, despite the many complexities of lockdowns and isolation, and found the time to talk to me in depth about their work. Without them, this book would not have come to fruition. Their names appear at the end of each chapter related to their specializations. In addition, I would like to thank my friend and academic partner, Prof. Sharon Snir, who takes the time to read what I write and help me think through the issues that arise.

I am grateful to the Emili Sagol Creative Arts Therapies Research Center at the University of Haifa of which I am a member, which has consistently provided me with the space and resources to accomplish the things that are important to me. In particular, I would like to thank Dr. Limor Goldner, who currently heads the research center, Danielle Friedlander, for her unwavering assistance, and Amit Pery, who is currently working with me on a project involving making videos of art therapists in their art therapy rooms in the education system. Thank you very much, all of you!

I would also like to express my appreciation to my publisher – Routledge (Taylor and Francis) – and especially Amanda Savage, my resourceful contact editor who can resolve everything and anything with talent.

Finally, I would like to thank my family: my parents Edna and Michael Neuberger, who gave me my curiosity and desire to understand things in depth, my beloved husband Alon, whose willingness and patience during the long days of writing are indeed extraordinary, and my lovely children, Maya, Inbal, Adi, and Shai, who take a real interest in their mother's writing. Your support and love enable me to keep on writing.

Art Therapy for Students with Learning Disabilities (LD) and Attention-Deficit/Hyperactivity Disorder (ADD/ADHD)

One

INTRODUCTION

This chapter deals with art therapy for students with learning disabilities (LD) and attention-deficit/hyperactivity disorder (ADD/ADHD). They are discussed together since the art therapists I interviewed have found that it is not always straightforward, especially when students are younger, to arrive at a diagnosis of LD, ADD/ADHD, or both. In addition, these two populations are similar in that they are born with a disability that impedes educational achievement. On the surface, this disability does not always appear to be associated with emotional problems. However, clinical experience shows that these students often accumulate an emotional burden from their encounters with environments that fail to acknowledge their specific needs. This emotional burden is not only expressed in class but also affects other areas of their lives.

Michal Bat-Or (2015) pointed out that these children's difficulties affect them in a variety of areas. At school, for example, they have problems paying attention in class, which impacts their relationships with their teachers and their academic achievement. During breaks, when they interact with other students, their impulsive behavior sometimes contributes to social problems and can escalate into quarrels and rejection. Within the family, these children often challenge their parents on issues related to discipline and setting boundaries, which can lead to tensions and friction. In contrast, ADD students (without the component of hyperactivity) are often lost when they disconnect from their environment. In the United States, over one-third of all children diagnosed with ADD/ADHD were reported to have high levels of emotional problems (Wehmeier et al., 2010). A European study clearly showed that children and adolescents with ADD/ADHD had more emotional problems as measured by the Strengths and Difficulties Questionnaire than children and adolescents without ADD/ADHD

DOI: 10.4324/9781003156918-1

(Coghill et al., 2006). Maor (1999) indicated that students with LD live in the same culture, have the same needs, and go through the same stages of development as their non-LD peers. However, they face obstacles and pressures that other children do not experience. These undermine their adaptability and contribute to the manifestation of varying degrees of psychological problems. Specifically, children with LD are characterized by difficulties in social information processing, low interpersonal skills, high levels of social rejection and loneliness, mood swings and depression, and internalizing and externalizing adjustment issues (Freilich & Shechtman, 2010).

The interviewees who contributed to this chapter all stated that it is difficult to differentiate LD from ADD/ADHD and that often both characteristics are combined. In some cases, parents may not be sure for a long period of time what is wrong with their children, which affects both the parents' and their offspring's stress and anxiety. Beyond their learning difficulties, these children experience the world differently and often accumulate emotional difficulties and other problems as a result of inadequate contact with their environment, which explains their need for psychotherapeutic treatment. One of their key difficulties is self-regulation, which makes it difficult for these children to function even in elementary school and causes them to engage in inappropriate social interactions. In addition, many of these students have language problems, so they find the verbal channel difficult to trust or use for communication. On the other hand, many of the therapists interviewed here highlighted the creativity of these students and noted that their artistic abilities were often more developed than other students. These children are difficult to reach in the usual way, but clearly the educational system needs to find a way to do so. Art therapy, because it is non-verbal, may constitute an important form of assistance.

THE THERAPEUTIC GOALS OF ART THERAPY

There are several key goals to art therapy with these students. Both the literature and the interviewees emphasized the value of art therapy in improving the self-image and self-confidence of these students (Maor, 1999). These students experience many moments of frustration in their lives in general and at school in particular. Sometimes one of the objectives is to encourage students to simply agree to work with art materials. Some students are afraid of recurrent experiences of failure and at times art is also seen as an experience where they can fail. One of the interviewees stated that art therapy provides "therapy through love"; in other words, that it reflects an admiring container back to them, to give these students the feeling that it is pleasant to be with them and that they can achieve success.

The interviewees also underscored the value of art therapy in connecting to the client's inner world and contents. This connection is often indirect and transits through characters from the content worlds that interest the student. This content often includes themes of distress and rescue, and an inability to save the protagonist. One of the therapists mentioned the goal of making connections between parts of experiences and different contents.

Given LD and ADD/ADHD students' difficulties in verbal communication, art therapy can also help them to express their emotions nonverbally (Freilich & Shechtman, 2010; Maor, 1999). The interviewees noted that the challenge often lies in finding the right material to help the students get involved in the work process. One interviewee mentioned that some students experience flooding, where it is difficult to stop, even for a moment. In such cases, the main goal is to learn just to be and to delve into work through the art materials.

Another factor relates to the use of art therapy, the art materials, and the therapeutic relationship to develop reflective observation. Safran (2003) argued that art therapy can be used reflectively to explore clients' symptoms, such as impulsivity in ADD/ADHD, because the artworks are the visual expression of and testimony to their emotional challenges. Alongside reflective observation, the interviewees mentioned that art therapy can help clients build their self-identity as students who are faced with specific difficulties and be better able to differentiate which problems are related to LD or ADD/ADHD and which are not.

Art therapy can also lead to progress in areas related to the disability itself. For example, one of the goals mentioned in the literature is to improve motor-perceptual functions. When these functions improve, so does the motivation to learn (Maor, 1999). Art therapy can encourage students with ADD/ADHD to be attentive to their inner rhythms and understand how different stimuli cause change (Murphy et al., 2004). Art therapy can provide a setting in which they can use diverse processing strategies to control behavior, while creating and strengthening their sense of control and regulation (Bat-Or, 2015; Murphy et al., 2004).

Since these students often also experience difficulties on the interpersonal level, art therapy can be used to improve social functioning (Maor, 1999). These students sometimes find it difficult to connect with other students and adults. Art therapy in an individual or group setting can provide a safe space for examining these relational issues. Some of the interviewees discussed improving the relationship with the student's family as well. In art therapy, students learn to express themselves and by extension can better express what they need in their family relationships. In cases where it is also possible to work with the parents, the goal is to improve the relationship and communication between family members.

Finally, one of the interviewees pointed to the importance of art therapy within the school system as a place where these students can vent, rest, and relax. Specifically, in schools where these students are forced to struggle with tasks that are very difficult for them throughout the day, art therapy can be experienced as a place where things are done differently, there are no academic requirements, and they can gather renewed strength.

CHALLENGES

The interviewees made it clear that one of the main challenges, especially in older students, is encouraging them in general to get into art therapy. Due to their past experiences, they often find it difficult to trust adults or give themselves a chance to be in a new relationship. It is important to help them understand that even though the treatment takes place at school, it is not about learning. In addition, transitions are sometimes problematic for these students. This can be seen in therapeutic sessions in the transition between activities (Murphy et al., 2004) as well as the transition from the classroom to the art therapy room and back, which can be complex. The rules in each framework are very different and students are required to adjust their behavior accordingly.

The structure of the art therapy session usually includes both art making with different materials and verbal reflections. Many interviewees said that they are not always able to involve their clients in creative processes. Some mentioned that they also keep games, therapeutic cards, or even a punching bag in the room, so that other activities can take place. Other therapists discussed these students' difficulties in listening to the art therapist during the verbal sharing after the artwork. This difficulty is magnified in group art therapy, where students must listen to others in the group (Murphy et al., 2004).

Sometimes, it is difficult for students to stay for the full hour of therapy. Their limited attention span also affects their ability to persevere on a creative process. Sometimes the art therapist will deliberately choose short experiences that can provide a sense of accomplishment. Students with LD and ADD/ADHD may also have physical difficulties working with certain art materials. The interviewees described situations in which artwork was torn, spilled, or disintegrated. In addition, the creativity and imagination in these students can engender vast fantasies which are then frustrated by their inability to render them technically in their artwork.

The interviewees drew attention to the very high associativity of these students. They sometimes enter the room flooded with stimuli. It is not easy for them to stop, to be, even at the level of discourse at the beginning of a session to say how they are feeling. In addition, clients may not know what they want to do in the session. Because these children have been so tightly managed over the years, they sometimes find it difficult to voice their own wishes or express their identity as a whole. One interviewee talked about how hard it is as an art therapist to choose the right words to say in the session. She felt that for these students, words are either invasive or condemning and describe something wrong. On the one hand, she is aware of these clients' heightened sensitivity since they often face stigma, but she also recognizes the difficulties associated with verbal communication which these students perceive as an unfriendly medium. Many interviewees said that in other contexts such as walking in the countryside or playing outside the therapy room, things could be expressed that were difficult to say in the room.

One of the interviewees specifically discussed students with ADD/ADHD under medication. Her view was that the differences between a student who took his or her medication and the same student on a day he or she had not, could be dramatic and impact the therapeutic relationship considerably. Some students benefit from medication because their attention span is longer. Others, according to her, lose their vitality, their ability to express themselves, and their creativity.

Some of the interviewees referred to their difficulties as art therapists. They described the existential difficulty of the therapeutic sessions and their fatigue by the end of the session. The need to adjust to the pace and transitions of the clients, which is especially difficult with students who are also hyperactive, is not easy, even for experienced therapists.

INTERVENTION TECHNIQUES AND DEDICATED WORKING MODELS

Emotional expression and reflection

Students with LD as well as students with ADD/ADHD often accumulate anger and frustration resulting from their years of complex interactions with the environment. Art therapy can help express these difficult feelings through work with clay, carpentry, papier maché, etc. (Bat-Or, 2015). After the emotional expression associated with working with the art materials, students can observe the processes reflectively. In this way, they learn about their conduct and the world around them (Bat-Or, 2015). This process also helps them to connect the verbal parts of the session to the nonverbal components and how they come together into one complete experience.

Bartoe (2014) surveyed art therapists in the United States on the most effective forms of intervention in treating children with ADD/ADHD. Most of them cited painting, drawing, sculpting, and collage. Painting can help achieve emotional regulation. Drawing can help maintain attention span and end the activity with a sense of accomplishment. Sculpture can be a way of emotionally expressing and expanding the client's attention span through 3D work. Collage allows for the expression of a wide range of emotions including aggression through the tearing of images. In addition, clients can integrate images from their daily life as well as their aspirations and thoughts about the future.

Building experiences of success

Art therapy can help begin to build experiences of success for these students who have faced failures so often in the past. Maor (1999) argued that the art therapist needs to help the client find an expressive channel in which s/he can excel and succeed. Learning to work with a particular material or technique and creating satisfying and admired products can help students transition to more positive feelings. The interviewees addressed both the importance of providing diverse choices to these students and also the many positive reinforcements provided throughout the work process. They stressed the importance of technical assistance, especially for students who are either awkward or find it difficult to put their creative ideas into practice.

Working on the concept of the "self"

Both populations can benefit from the work in art therapy on the concept of the "self" or different aspects of the "self", and the way in which they are expressed using art materials. Since these students often experience low self-esteem, thinking about the types of "self" they want to develop, and those types they would less like to develop can help shape more positive self-perception (Bat-Or, 2015).

Strengthening sensorimotor functions

The contact with the art materials, the work and the experience with them, allows the student to feel, process, and reinforce sensorimotor functions. Cutting, tearing, kneading, rolling, squeezing, and working with various drawing tools can improve fine motor skills, eye-hand coordination, and graphomotor performance (Maor, 1999). Safran (2003) emphasized the importance of finding art materials that activate various levels of bodily engagement. She noted that sensory-oriented materials such as scented markers can engage children and serve as an opportunity to assess their distractibility when stimulated on a sensory level.

Constructing the work environment and the therapeutic session

Bat-Or (2015) emphasized the need to construct the client's work environment, especially for students with ADD/ADHD. This involves setting up specific work areas for art making in different materials and organizing the work process with the client by jointly adhering to the work stages. One of the interviewees suggested preparing separate baskets containing different sets of art materials. Another interviewee mentioned the importance of not putting out all the art materials, but rather choosing them to reflect the student's needs and to avoid flooding. This therapist also described how she structures the therapeutic session. The first part is composed of the emotional discourse based on techniques such as cards. This part focuses on building listening and reciprocity abilities. The second part is more creative, open, and free, but the art therapist selects which art materials are best suited to each student.

Group therapy to improve social functioning

There is considerable literature on group art therapy especially for students with ADD/ADHD, but also for students with LD. Reddy and Alperin (2016) argued that within the group setting, students can begin to observe their own behaviors and feelings and those of others toward them. Safran (2003) recommended dividing sessions with ADD/ADHD students into three main parts: repeating the rules and key contents from the previous session, creating with art materials, and finally, group sharing. Murphy et al. (2004) also described group art therapy for children with ADD/ADHD, which was set up because it was difficult for these children to be integrated into other groups. The therapeutic session was divided into three parts, each consisting of a different activity: (1) Movement activity for the whole group where the ideas for the activity come from within the group itself, followed by sitting in a circle and sharing the feelings elicited by the activity; (2) Free work in art materials followed by a presentation of the products to the group members; (3) A concluding and relaxing activity to help students return to life outside the art therapy room. The group met for seven months for 1.5 hours each week. The authors emphasized the importance specifically for this population of maintaining a regular schedule to create external boundaries within which a freer expression of emotions is possible. To help the students be attentive to each other, the therapists used a symbolic microphone that the students passed to each other so that only the one holding it was allowed to speak.

The interviewees here also addressed the process of selecting students for the group. Given the range of difficulties in this population, they emphasized how important it is to get to know the students and make sure that group work is indeed appropriate in terms of work goals, the students' energy levels, degree of cooperation, special problems, etc. They recommended limiting the number of participants to create a group that feels comfortable and allows the art therapist to feel in control. Sometimes it is possible to integrate students with similar difficulties from different classes and even from different age groups. The group sessions are designed to provide an opportunity to be in touch with other students who are coping with similar difficulties. One of the interviewees said that she tries to form groups of three students, where only one has a social difficulty. She has found this format to be useful in enabling the students to examine their patterns of relationships with others.

The interviewees described a variety of ways of working together. One stated that she asks the students how they would like the group to work; for example, each week someone else can lead the session, or the students can decide together how to work, or the art therapist directs the session. Another interviewee implements a three-part session. In the first part, the students are asked how they are doing, which is designed to teach them to look at themselves and link sessions. In the second part, they discuss what will be done during the session and the art therapist describes how she sees the division of roles in the group. Then they work with the art materials. The third part is a summary that includes an observation of what was in the session and how it relates to the whole process. Students are invited to exhibit the artworks they made during the session and learn to observe and respond to the works of others. The third interviewee emphasized the importance of letting each student work individually and that the decision to work together could come from the students but is not obligatory. In particular in the education system where everyone usually progresses at a uniform pace, the process and the personal pace of each student in the group are meaningful. The fourth interviewee emphasized finding a theme for each group. She described a group, for example, that focused on the issue of self-advocacy that is so important to these students. In another group, the students compiled a visual diary. In each session, they worked on a page in a different material and at the end of the year, the pages were turned into one diary testifying to their shared experience.

The interviewees also discussed a group-class art therapy model that is often used in Israel (Ofer Yarom et al., 2021). In this model, which applies to special education classes, the art therapist works with a whole class, including the teacher and the assistant. This enables observations that the homeroom teacher and the art therapist can use to think about specific students and understand them better. The group-class therapy session should ideally be followed by a weekly hour where the team meets to process the experience and get supervision from the art therapist. One of the interviewees described working with songs in this format. In each session, one student chooses and presents a different song to the class, and the creative work is related to the song. The goal is first and foremost to give each student the opportunity to be the center of the group. Another goal is for the other members of the group to relate to the song and discover something about their classmate in the process.

The open studio model

The interviewees also discussed the advantages of the open studio model (Heller, 2021) for these students. The idea of an open studio can be especially successful when it contains aspects of integration. One interviewee described a model in which classroom teachers can integrate students with LD and ADD/ADHD with other students in an open studio. Each class had several spots available in the open studio each week, and the students took turns taking part. This particular open studio ended up being composed of two-thirds permanent students and one-third students who took turns. In the studio, new interactions were formed around the artworks and the art materials. The teacher and the art therapist ran the studio together. At the beginning of each session, the students gathered. Then, they could move between art materials, choose and work. The art therapist and the teacher provided technical help. At the end of the session, there were a few minutes for cleanup and transitioning back to the school space. Each session lasted 45 minutes but could be extended for those students who wanted to continue. Another interviewee talked about the importance of warm up and wind down in the open studio context. When students first come to the studio, they may not know what they want to do. In such situations, she tries not to solve the problem for them, but lets them wander around, touch, experiment with materials, and decide for themselves which material appeals to them. At the end of the session, the cleanup contributes to a sense of construction and organization that is important to impart to these students. The works can then be grouped for phenomenological observation or to choose a word that describes feelings in relation to the artwork.

Parent–child art psychotherapy

In recent years, the Israel Ministry of Education has begun to apply a parent–child art psychotherapy model in kindergartens and schools (Regev & Tamir, 2021). In these cases, parents are invited for a weekly therapeutic session at school or in kindergarten. One of the interviewees noted that she sometimes asks the parents to attend a parent–child art psychotherapy session for a certain part of the treatment, especially in cases where she feels that the student's disabilities or difficulties affect the parent–child relationship. This can be manifested in multiple conflicts between the child and one or both parents, or in situations where one parent avoids contact or finds it difficult to be with the child. She at times invites several dyads to work together. For example, she organized a session for a group of three fathers and their children to do carpentry together, in which each third session was devoted to parental guidance for both parents together. Another interviewee said that she divides these dyadic sessions into a more structured part guided by her and an open part where parent and child choose what they want to do in the room.

Working together with the art therapist

Furneaux-Blick (2019) described her joint creative process with a girl with LD. She suggested that working on a joint activity strengthened the therapeutic relationship by enabling non-verbal communication to take place. Alongside this strengthening, there was a shared experience of being together, which in turn provided a more fertile terrain for countertransference to occur. Countertransference enabled Furneaux-Blick to recognize how a child with LD feels.

Combining mindfulness and guided imagery with art therapy

Mindfulness can also be combined with art therapy. Sin (2017) reported that students with ADD/ADHD can benefit from mindfulness-based interventions in art therapy for individuals in need of emotional regulation. Interventions such as encouraging the sensory exploration of art materials can promote awareness and discussions about the sensations, thoughts, and feelings that were elicited, which the individual became aware of during the process. One of the interviewees described the use of mindfulness and guided imagery at the beginning of therapeutic sessions. In her view, for students who are not hyperactive, imagining a quiet place can be very helpful. By contrast, hyperactive students sometimes find it hard to imagine being in a quiet place, thus making this exercise less suitable for them.

Playing and experimenting with materials

Some of the interviewees described these students' attraction to exploratory contact with materials. One interviewee depicted a student who was playing with fire and candles to see what could melt and in what way. Another interviewee mentioned a girl who used Slime for many sessions and enclosed each one in a separate box. Each had different components from the others. At the start of each session, she would open all the boxes and examine her previous works before making a new Slime. The art therapist suggested that the Slime, which included transformation, touch, and attempts to use the material to its maximum, helped this student test her own boundaries non-verbally through the material.

Pottery

Shahak (2012) found that ADD/ADHD individuals reported positive changes in the way they conducted themselves and their ability to cope with ADD/ADHD in their daily lives by working with pottery. Her findings indicated that the dynamic ongoing creative processes, which were structured according to different work stages defined at a varying times, places, and rhythms, helped them deal with their difficulties. For example, circular wheel work involves learning the clay throwing technique and developing skills to make pieces of pottery to exhibit or even sell. Each of these stages has a therapeutic value and contributes to the students' ability to control, defer gratification, organize and plan, effective time management, focus and awareness, mental clarity, development of inner speech, self-regulation, self-expression, strengthening self-confidence, and encouraging acceptance and self-esteem.

Wood

The interviewees referred to the benefits of building things out of wood. Sawing, hammering, and gluing with hot glue appeal to this population. This type of activity practices regulation, the mastery of the material, and can produce a strong sense of success. One of the interviewees said that she equipped the art therapy room with a variety of woodworking tools and suggested that the practical nature of woodworking (for example, building a chair), attracts many students. Each client chooses what s/he wants to do, and the work at least in the early stages takes place with the help of the art therapist (for safety reasons). Sawing together, for instance, provides a shared experience and also a kind of to and fro reminiscent of the infantile rhythms in the mother–baby relationship and requires reciprocity. In addition, parent and child can be invited to work with wood together. Wood is a hard material, but it can be combined with both soft and ready-made materials. One of the interviewees mentioned that clients often wanted to make an object that moved, such as a spinning wheel or another part that could move. Safety precautions are essential when working with wood. These works can be taken home (after displaying them to admiring classmates) and are often a source of pride on the part of the students.

Plaster

A number of interviewees noted that plaster can be used to create a satisfying shape and product relatively quickly. One interviewee said that sometimes students like to make plaster casts for their "broken" arms or legs, perhaps symbolically to represent something that may be perceived as broken in them. Symbolically, plaster is a material that makes pieces whole and can be seen as a material that forms a second skin or can be placed in a mold. One interviewee invites clients to think of a character from the movies or TV shows or computer games. The characters they choose often have enormous symbolic meaning. For example, one student chose a character that explodes when approached. The art therapist helps the students build a wire skeleton of the figure and then coat it with strips of plaster. The dried figure can be painted and objects in its environment can also be made. The character can be discussed, especially when the meaning is highly relevant to the client. These works can also be taken home and students are often very proud of them.

Spray paint

One of the interviewees described using spray paint for 3D work and for graffiti tags and all kinds of signs. There is something in the splash of color, in working on large surfaces, and in the need for control and regulation that is very appropriate for this particular population. Spray painting should only be done in a well-ventilated room or outside.

Filament (hot wire) for Styrofoam cutting

One interviewee described the use of filament to cut Styrofoam to make specific shapes or simply to cut pieces. Cutting requires a certain rhythm that cannot be accelerated. She reported that students with ADD/ADHD manage to concentrate and cut at the pace of the filament and that they experienced considerable satisfaction from the mastery of cutting and using these tools. Safety precautions are required.

Textiles

Some of the interviewees, especially those working with adolescents, sometimes suggest knitting, embroidery, or macrame. For these students, the growth of the project over time helps to connect different sessions into one complete experience. The contact with soft materials is experienced as soothing and regulating.

THE MEANING OF ART

The interviewees all emphasized that the primary purpose of art materials for these students is to enable them to experience success. After years of struggles and failures, especially within the school setting, experiences of success with art materials are very important and empowering. One of the art therapists emphasized that she allows students to take the artworks home, and show them to their families, to experience more admiration and appreciation of their efforts.

Importantly, art materials can constitute an alternative mode of expression for individuals who find verbal communication difficult. By using art materials, they can express a wide range of emotions non-verbally (Murphy et al., 2004). When words cannot express feelings and thoughts, art expresses their creativities and abilities and can at times form the bridge to convey these experiences verbally.

Finally, the use of art materials helps strengthen the functions that are weak in these students. For example, with respect to students with ADD/ADHD, Hinz (2009) argued that sensory-oriented materials such as clay, watercolor, and acrylic paint can help focus and sustain focus because they can orient attention exclusively to sensation in the here-and-now.

COLLABORATIVE INTERVENTIONS INVOLVING PARENTS AND STAFF MEMBERS

Working with parents

The interviewees noted that parents of LD and ADD/ADHD children find it difficult to attend the three parental guidance meetings recommended by the Ministry of Education. When the children are younger, parents are still processing their child's difficulties and often need to cope with their anger, denial, and loss of trust in the system. As the children grow older, parents tend to believe that after multiple meetings they are unlikely to hear anything new. This is one of the reasons why efforts to get parents to come to meetings and an emphasis on the student's strengths are so important. At the same time, one of the interviewees noted the importance of acknowledging the student's problems in conversations with parents and cautioned that splits, where the teacher is perceived as bad and the art therapist as good, should be avoided. What is crucial is to work collaboratively to help the student progress.

These meetings with the parents call for a great deal of acceptance and support and an attempt to be empathetic with respect to their situation. On the other hand, it is important to help them look at their child from a broader perspective and deal with less obvious issues. For example, one interviewee argued that it is not always easy for parents to connect their child's difficulties to his or her social problems, thus making it crucial to help them see how their child's characteristics affect his or her interactions with other people. Bat-Or (2015) discussed parental observation of the artworks their child has done during art therapy as part of parental guidance (with the child's consent). Viewing the artworks can help them understand their child's personal experiences as a student.

Working with staff members

The interviewees noted that even in regular classrooms, the staff needs to be informed of the emotional difficulties faced by LD and ADD/ADHD students. Teachers need to understand the functions of the art therapist and how to contact him/her when needed. During staff meetings, theoretical material on art therapy and even case studies can be presented so that teachers can understand what the art therapist does. Some of the interviewees also mentioned informal meetings during school breaks or on the phone, in which important conversations about students in therapy can take place. One of the interviewees said that she tries to be available in situations when one of her students experiences a crisis in school. Her presence promotes the relationship with both student and teacher and conveys the message that even in difficult times, they can be together and move on and sometimes even talk about it in the art therapy room. These are anxious situations that can lead to splits and it is precisely the joint presence that helps the student calm down and mobilize forces.

The interviewees argued that in regular schools, unlike in special education, there is still not enough teamwork that enables close contact between the class teacher and the art therapist. These regular meetings can contribute considerably to the students' well-being. They stated that they often approach teachers in the staff room, make an effort to get to know the educators and homeroom teachers, and sometimes try to mediate and convey messages that can help their clients conduct themselves better in the classroom. They also try to reflect the stronger and more successful facets of the students, which can be better seen in activities that do not involve academic assignments.

One of the interviewees specifically addressed the transitions in the school between the art therapy room and outside it. She described a student who, after years of working in art therapy, chose to study art and wanted her final project to present some of the content that had preoccupied her over the years. In a careful work process, which involved collaboration between the art therapist and the art teacher, the student was helped to make decisions about what content to reveal and what to leave private in the art therapy room.

CLINICAL ILLUSTRATION

Dor was ten years old, and in the fourth grade, when he was referred to art therapy. He was the eldest son in a family of three children. His father worked as an engineer and his mother as a teacher. As early as kindergarten, difficulties began to emerge. He had problems sitting quietly and was in constant motion. Although he had some friends, he tended to react impulsively and sometimes even violently, which caused many children to avoid him. His parents reported that even at home, his conduct was complex. It was difficult to get him to kindergarten on time or go to bed in the evening. When Dor entered first grade, the problems got worse. Dor found it very difficult to sit in class and work on assignments and many times failed to keep up with the class or submit assignments on time. By the time Dor started attending art therapy sessions he had already experienced several difficult years of school. These experiences included repeated failures and a feeling of not being understood. Several attempts were made to try medication, with no visible improvement. His feeling of resentment became more and more ingrained.

Dor was not sure that attending art therapy sessions was right for him. When the art therapist came to class to call him, he hesitated. He was not sure he was willing to give a chance to anything else. He lumbered after the art therapist and sat down on a chair. His gaze was lowered, with his head sunk between his shoulders. He had a hard time noticing what was going on in the room. He began to spin in the chair in a desperate attempt to calm himself. The art therapist sat down next to him. She smiled. It was quiet for a moment. She told him a little about herself and suggested he could walk around the room to see what was in it. Dor agreed reluctantly.

They started walking around the room. The room had a variety of work areas set up: a work area near a table, a painting area on the wall, and a clay work area. Woodworking instruments hung in one corner. Dor looked up and glanced with interest at the saw and drill. "What can be done with that?" He asked and "Are you really allow to use it?". The art therapist smiled. She told him that the ideas were his and that she would be happy to help him build something. "Can I build whatever I want?" Dor thought he might not have understood correctly. "Yes", the art therapist answered. Slowly Dor looked at the planks and pieces of wood in a large box. In his mind, he had already built a boat that would take him far, far away from there. He placed the pieces on the table and wondered how to proceed. "What exactly do you want to make?" The art therapist asked. "A boat", he replied. "Can you draw me how you would like it to look?" Dor took a piece of paper and a pencil and began to draw, at first in weak thin lines and later with a more confident hand. The art therapist looked, asked a number of questions, and made a number of suggestions. Together they devised a work plan.

Dor came to the following sessions with joy and confidence. In class, he told his friends that he was building a boat in the art therapy room. Within therapy, he learned skill after skill. At first, he needed a lot of help and even gestures like sawing were done together with the art therapist; however, over time he became more and more independent. He learned how to operate the various tools, and how to decide which part to connect and where. He learned to organize the tools for work and also how to put everything back in place at the end of the session. Dor's difficulties did not cease, but he had a place where he could experience success, a place where he slowly also agreed to share his life outside the therapy room verbally with the art therapist. A few months later the boat was ready and when his father came to school to help him take it home, he was the proudest.

SUMMARY

Art therapy with students with LD and ADD/ADHD is primarily intended to raise the self-esteem and self-confidence of these students. In so doing, space is given to the expression of emotions and content that they sometimes find difficult to put in words. In art therapy, they learn to reflect on the difficulties that challenge them and their evolving identity. They also work to improve their motor-perceptual functions and processes of regulation and control. Some treatments also specifically address difficulties in interpersonal relationships with friends and family.

However, it is not always easy for these students to be in art therapy. They sometimes find it difficult to relate to or have trust in the therapeutic setting after the many frustrations in their lives. It is sometimes difficult for them to transition between the educational and therapeutic frameworks and also between activities within the session. Sometimes they find it difficult to create, sometimes to observe, and sometimes the very fact of staying put for a 45-minute session is experienced as challenging. There are clients who find it technically difficult to create or are so overwhelmed with stimuli that they have difficulty choosing what to do. Added to all this are changes in medications or variations in doses, which sometimes challenge the therapeutic relationship.

This chapter presented a wide range of alternatives for working with LD and ADD/ADHD students. These include constructing the therapeutic framework and focusing on working on the areas in which these students have difficulty. Settings such as group therapy, the open studio, and joint interventions with the art therapist or with parents can be used successfully. Numerous art materials and therapeutic interventions are beneficial for these students, as noted by the experienced art therapists interviewed here.

REFERENCES

Bartoe, H. L. (2014). *Art therapy and children with ADHD: A survey of art therapists* (A thesis submitted in partial fulfillment of the requirements for the degree of Master of Science in Psychology, Kaplan University).

Bat-Or, M. (2015). Art therapy with AD/HD children: Exploring possible selves via art. In E. E. Kourkoutas, A. Hart & A. Mouzaki (Eds.), *Innovative practice and interventions for children and adolescents with psychosocial difficulties, disorders, and disabilities* (pp. 373–389). Newcastle upon Tyne: Cambridge Scholar Publishing.

Coghill, D., Spiel, G., Baldursson, G., Dopfner, M., Lorenzo, M. J., Ralston et al. (2006). Which factors impact on clinician-rated impairment in children with ADHD? *European Child & Adolescent Psychiatry, 15*, 30–37.

Freilich, R., & Shechtman, Z. (2010). The contribution of art therapy to the social, emotional, and academic adjustment of children with learning disabilities. *The Arts in Psychotherapy, 37*, 97–105.

Furneaux-Blick, S. (2019). Painting together: How joint activity reinforces the therapeutic relationship with a young person with learning disabilities. *International Journal of Art Therapy, 24*(4), 169–180.

Heller, A. (2021). The "Open Studio" model in educational frameworks. In D. Regev & S. Snir (Eds.), *Integrating art therapy into education: A collective volume.* (pp. 111–127). Routledge (Taylor & Francis Group).

Hinz, L. D. (2009). *Expressive therapies continuum: A framework for using art in therapy.* Routledge (Taylor & Francis Group).

Maor, P. (1999). Art therapy for children with learning disabilities. *ISER: Issues in Special Education & Rehabilitation, 14*(1), 37–51. Retrieved October 15, 2020, from http://www.jstor.org/stable/23452530 (In Hebrew).

Murphy, J., Paisley, D., & Pardoe, L. (2004). An art therapy group for impulsive children. *International Journal of Art Therapy, 9*(2), 59–68.

Ofer Yarom, M. Court, D., & Shamir, A. (2021). ECRAB (An Emotional, Cognitive, Rehabilitative and Behavioral Model): Group-class arts therapy in a special education school. In D. Regev & S. Snir (Eds.), *Integrating art therapy into education: A collective volume.* (pp. 147–166). Routledge (Taylor & Francis Group).

Reddy, L. A., & Alperin, A. (2016). Children with attention-deficit/hyperactivity disorder. In C. Haen & S. Aronson (Eds.), Handbook of children and adolescent group therapy: A practitioner's reference (pp. 322–334). Routledge (Taylor & Francis Group).

Regev, D., & Tamir, R. (2021). Parent-child art psychotherapy in the education system. In D. Regev & S. Snir, (Eds.), Integrating art therapy into education: A collective volume. Routledge (Taylor & Francis Group).

Safran, D. S. (2003). An art therapy approach to attention-deficit/hyperactivity disorder. In C. A. Malchiodi (Ed.), Handbook of art therapy. Psychiatric services (pp. 181–192). The Guildford Press.

Shahak, H. (2012). The interaction between pottery and Attention Deficit Hyperactivity Disorder (ADHD). (Presented in Partial Fulfillment of the Requirements for the Degree of Master of Creative Arts Therapies, University of Haifa, Israel) (In Hebrew).

Sin, J. (2017). Mindfulness-based art therapy in working with school-aged children with ADHD in emotional regulation (Presented in Partial Fulfillment of the Requirements for the Degree of Master of Arts Concordia University Montreal, Quebec, Canada).

Wehmeier, P. M., Schacht, A., & Barkley, R. A. (2010). Social and emotional impairment in children and adolescents with ADHD and the impact on quality of life. Journal of Adolescent Health, 46, 209–217.

BRIEF BIOGRAPHIES OF THE ART THERAPISTS WHO CONTRIBUTED TO THIS CHAPTER

Merav Adler, art therapist (M.A.) and supervisor, has worked as a kindergarten teacher for many years and for eight years working in the education system as an art therapist with students with LD and ADD/ADHD in kindergarten and elementary school.

Merav Baram, art therapist (M.A.) and supervisor, lecturer at the School of Society, and the Arts at Ono Academic College, has worked for 22 years in the education system as an art therapist with students with LD and ADD/ADHD of all ages.

Neta Harari, art therapist (M.A.), has worked for seven years in the education system, including five years as an art therapist with adolescents with LD and ADD/ADHD.

Meital Harosh, art therapist and supervisor, studied educational psychology (M.A.), has worked for 12 years in the education system as an art therapist with students with LD and ADD/ADHD in elementary school.

Tamar Sade-Dor, art therapist (M.A.) and supervisor, has worked for 22 years in the education system, including 13 years as an art therapist with adolescents with LD and ADD/ADHD.

Miri Simonson, art therapist (M.A.) and supervisor, has worked as an occupational therapist for many years in the education system and 12 years working in the education system as an art therapist with students with LD and ADD/ADHD in kindergarten and elementary school.

Hadas Tamir, art therapist (M.A.) and supervisor, has worked for eight years in the education system, including six years as an art therapist with adolescents with LD and ADD/ADHD.

Two

INTRODUCTION

This chapter deals with art therapy for students who are deaf or hard of hearing (D/HH). It is worth noting at the outset of this chapter that the interviewees all emphasized the diversity of this population. To understand this diversity in depth, it is crucial to indicate that today, given the advances in technology that can improve hearing through a cochlear implant, parents can decide on surgery for their children at a young age, which restores hearing. However, an implant in itself is not enough, and all these children must go through a process of hearing rehabilitation, which depends to a great extent on the recruitment of the family circle to the process.

The interviewees defined a number of categories of students with D/HH. The first is composed of students whose mother, father, or both are D/HH. These families often do not want implants and feel that there is no reason to "fix" their children because nothing is wrong with them. In these families, the students tend to mix with many other D/HH people so there is less of a sense of exception. The second category is composed of D/HH students who have hearing parents. These two categories break down into numerous subcategories based on level of hearing, the success of the implant surgery, family support during the rehabilitation process, the association of D/HH with additional disabilities, and integration into regular or special education. This chapter focuses on students with a range of characteristics who are in various stages of coping with D/HH.

King (2020) referred to the difference between deaf and Deaf. She argued that those who define themselves with a small letter refer primarily to the medical model and emphasize the auditory condition and mode of communication. In contrast, those who define themselves with a capital letter refer to a mode of existence that reflects

DOI: 10.4324/9781003156918-2

the cultural aspect of anyone who was born deaf or became deaf in childhood, whether exposed to deaf culture or not. The interviewees all addressed the issue of the deaf community and stated that it is easy for students born to D/HH families to belong to this community. By contrast, students born to hearing families may only connect to this community at later stages in their lives, if ever.

In general, for most D/HH students, the main difficulty centers on issues of communication and language. Eye contact and facial expressions are critical factors in making contact. To remain in the relationship, the art therapist must find a way to make contact in the client's way through sign language, pantomime, gestures, facial expressions, spoken language, or a combination of all the above. In addition, the art therapist must use vocabulary that is comprehensible to the client and is part of his/her world of concepts. Sometimes, communication difficulties can lead to inaccurate over-diagnosis and/or under-diagnosis of emotional difficulties in these students. Hoggard (2006) argued that an art therapist who is about to work with this population should have a robust grasp of the meaning of difficulties in communication and language and the impact of these difficulties on building a therapeutic relationship. It is worth pointing out that there is a difference between the sign language of the hearing (Manual English Signed System), which actually signifies the words spoken, and the sign language of the deaf community. This language has evolved over the years and has its own syntactic features, which do not correspond to the syntax of verbal language. This language also varies as a function of the geographic location, the age of the user, and the degree of formality of the situation. Most of the interviewees stated that although they had worked with this population for many years and recognized the importance of using sign language, they were not proficient enough.

D/HH children look the same as other children and have the same cognitive abilities as hearing children: they walk, laugh, cry, and have the same basic needs. However, D/HH children do not have the same language skills to express themselves and most experience difficulties receiving and processing aural (spoken) communication (Boyle & Snow, 2019). In addition, because the majority population is hearing, and because 95% of D/HH children are born into systems (i.e., family and community) that know little or nothing about Deaf culture or are not proficient in sign language, children can experience feelings of isolation and loneliness, as well as other emotional challenges related to interacting with the world (Tapia-Fuselier & Ray, 2019). Boyle and Snow (2019) emphasized that D/HH students may perceive themselves as different if they have hearing problems or difficulty communicating with others, especially if they wear cochlear implants/ hearing aids. These difficulties can lead to their referral to art therapy.

A number of interviewees felt that these students' sense of space is impaired, and some may find it difficult for them to locate where someone is situated or who is approaching them. The result can be restlessness and heightened vigilance to the environment. Other interviewees stated that precisely because of the use of sign language, which is three-dimensional, these students may have a more acute understanding of space than hearing students and can orient themselves well in it.

The interviewees drew attention to these students' difficulties using abstract concepts. Early theory and practice assumed that D/HH children were less able to reason abstractly. These assumptions may have stemmed from the fact that D/HH often places children in situations where they are not exposed to abstract concepts. It is now clear that D/HH individuals have abstract thinking skills but need opportunities to develop them. The ability to manipulate abstract concepts depends on both the level of communication and the way their immediate environment deals with D/HH.

The difficulties faced by students with D/HH, especially those from hearing families, who sometimes experience loneliness and a sense they do not belong, can also lead to issues of social stigma, rejection, or poor engagement with peers. The interviewees noted that these students sometimes find it hard to connect with classmates, especially with hearing peers. One interviewee stated that adolescent clients often begin to be aware that it is difficult for them to engage in social interactions. When the social framework involves groups, they tend to miss important information and find it hard to take part in a conversation or joint activities.

Studies conducted in recent years indicate that there are also differences in pictorial characteristics between the artistic output of D/HH and hearing individuals. Lev-Wiesel and Yosipov-Kaziav (2005) found that figure paintings of D/HH individuals were significantly different from the figure paintings of hearing people in terms of a number of body parts depicted such as ears, eyes, mouth, nose, hands and arms, body contours, and eyebrows. Studies have noted differences in emphasis on the ears given the importance that D/HH individuals attach to this significant organ in their lives. Another study in which I took part (Avrahami-Winaver et al., 2020) compared the family drawings of D/HH children and their hearing parents to those of hearing children and their parents. Significant differences were found with respect to a number of pictorial phenomena including the representation of objects reminiscent of hearing aids (such as seashells or more abstract forms) within the family pictorial space.

THE THERAPEUTIC GOALS OF ART THERAPY

Hoggard (2006) argued that one of the main goals of art therapy with D/HH students is to allow them to express experiences and feelings that are sometimes difficult for them to convey in words. The realm of art therapy makes non-verbal expression possible, which is highly appropriate for these students and can lessen levels of anxiety and depression (Boyle & Snow, 2019). In art therapy, the product emerging from work with the art materials within the therapeutic context reflects the mental processes that take place in therapy and forms the basis of the therapeutic work. In addition, art can become a means of expression when students feel it is hard to bridge the communication gap between themselves and their hearing parents (Horovitz, 2007). One interviewee suggested that the notion of privacy does not always exist for these students. Sometimes this is the first setting where they encounter a non-judgmental other who accepts diverse forms of expression. In the art therapy room, people can talk about their fears and can express themselves freely.

Another goal of art therapy is to mediate between the different worlds in the student's life: between the world of D/HH people and the world of hearing people, between what "I understand" and what "I do not understand". Within the therapeutic relationship, the desire to understand and be understood is reciprocal. On the one hand, there is the client's need to be understood and on the other hand, the therapist's need for the client to understand him/her as well. When the therapist acknowledges the issue of communication, which engages both, the client's experience is legitimated and normalized.

Another goal is to raise the self-esteem of these students. The wide range of art materials made available to them, and the opportunity to make personal art products enable them to feel they can succeed and can prompt these students to discover their strengths (Boyle & Snow, 2019). The interviewees often remarked that in the school setting, where these students often struggle to succeed and progress, the chance to create an impressive art product can enormously enhance their self-esteem.

Art therapy can also contribute to thinking and using abstract concepts. Working with art materials provides experiences in abstract thinking through concepts such as conservation, sequential ordering, grouping of objects, and spatial relationships (Boyle & Snow, 2019). One interviewee noted that the commonplace question "How do you feel?" is not an obvious one for some students with D/HH, since they are not often asked. In art therapy, the client is invited to work from sensory experiences and slowly move toward answering this question more broadly.

Many interviewees noted that D/HH students find it hard to make decisions. This may at times stem from the fact that their family and educational circles typically make choices for them out of a desire to help and protect them. The interviewees indicated that through exposure to multiple experiences, these students slowly learn what options are available to them and learn to exercise the choice process. Questions such as "Which do you prefer?", "What do you want to work on?", "What makes you feel good?", "What field do you want to work in?", and "What do you want?" are very important questions for personal exploration and joint work.

As these students grow older, they begin to deal with their sense of difference with respect to the general population. This is more noticeable in children of hearing parents, especially when there are not strong enough ties to the deaf community. In such cases, some of the goals will be self-determination and an attempt to observe their identity as a person with D/HH.

Finally, the interviewees also referred to the importance of social integration. They noted that many D/HH students feel very lonely. The interviewees stressed the importance of helping them make contact with hearing students since at times they feel they are not understood both linguistically and otherwise. This feeling is particularly important in the classroom where these students have the opportunity to interact with hearing students. In this respect, the goal is to teach students to connect with others in a way that takes their needs and other students' needs into account. In addition, these students should be helped to learn to engage in more complex interactions with their peers.

CHALLENGES

While working in art therapy, D/HH students cannot engage in art making and use sign language at the same time. This split, in which the client has to choose whether to be within the artwork or within communication, is something these clients are familiar with since childhood (Hoggard, 2006). Sometimes their body language conveys what they cannot say during the creative work. It is important for the art therapist to be attentive to this form of communication. In addition, art therapists need to stand or sit in a place where clients can see them well, even while creating. This way, they can communicate with them when needed. The interviewees noted that all students, including those with a cochlear implant, rely on lip reading, which should thus be facilitated by the physical positioning of the therapist.

Some of the interviewees mentioned that the clients did not have sufficient opportunities to develop certain areas of knowledge. This difficulty is not limited to abstract concepts. One interviewee indicated that they sometimes have "black holes" on issues that no one has ever bothered to talk to them about. These can sometimes be very, very trivial issues that have somehow been neglected and not properly mediated. For example, this therapist described a client with high abilities, who was discovered in high school that he did not know his mother's first name. It had never come up for discussion, no one ever asked him, and he did not know that she could be called anything else than "Mom". Another interviewee mentioned that these children may not know to be wary of strangers. Perhaps due to over-protection or incomplete communication of ideas, she was surprised to find that it was not clear to them that, for example, they must not go off with a stranger simply because s/he offers them candies.

The interviewees also referred to the language barrier. When clients use sign language efficiently and the art therapists do not, this creates a disparity that is sometimes difficult to bridge. It is evident that the use of sign language is now less of a need than in the past, since most students with cochlear implants are able to hear or read lips at some level. This may also be the reason why most of the art therapists I interviewed said they were not completely fluent in sign language despite multiple years of working with students from this population. One of the interviewees said that when she started to work with this population, she felt very different because she did not know sign language. To this day her vocabulary is limited, and she seeks the help of her clients. She tells clients that just as they have problems with oral language and hearing, she has problems with sign language.

One of the interviewees referred to the time it takes clients to learn the language of art. In her view, the process of learning a new language is not always straightforward for D/HH students and it often takes time to experience each art material, until they can actually use it for purposes of emotional expression. Another interviewee also referred to the pace of therapy and said that it is generally slower since it takes these students longer to process the emerging content and transfer it between different languages (art, oral, and sign) to achieve a full understanding.

INTERVENTION TECHNIQUES AND DEDICATED WORKING MODELS

Setting the scene

Hoggard (2006) noted that the way D/HH students create is different from that of other students. In order to allow them to express their experiences, the art therapist must understand that they need sufficient time to create the environment in which the event they want to represent took place. The gradual construction of the scene gives them the space to share their experiences. In almost all of the interviews, the art therapists addressed the need of clients with D/HH to produce a scene from their lives and invite the art therapist with them into it. Some of them often worked with plasticine because it can be used to model a situation concretely and breathe life into the characters in the story. In this way, the clients are able to depict events from their lives non-verbally. The art therapist can offer extensions of material use or a combination of materials or extensions of the scene and its surroundings. In the same context, one of the art therapists also mentioned working in a sandbox. While using miniatures in the sandbox, clients can build a situation and sometimes even invite her to take part in the story.

To work with the students' difficulties making choices, the interviewees suggested that a wide range of potential experiences be made available to them. These experiences are specific to each client and can include any aspect of the work from learning to use a pencil or drawing self-portraits to sensory experiences with the art materials. The important thing is to experience the use of power, and what it is like to get dirty, and all types of experiences they may not have had. The variety, experiences and possibilities, enables these students to choose what suits them best for self-expression.

The process of learning the language of art can unfold in a variety of ways. Sometimes, simply presenting the art material is sufficient but other times the art therapist needs to demonstrate the affordance of each material. One of the art therapists described how a client learned to work with watercolors. They sat together, each with a sheet of paper, and made different playful attempts. These included lifting the page and seeing what happens to the color when it drips. Another interviewee, who works with kindergarten children, said that expanding art-making possibilities is not always straightforward since these children sometimes tend to stick with a certain art material, they feel safe with, and are afraid to try other things. She experiments with all sorts of ways to offer them more diverse exposure to art materials and techniques.

Creating and observing

Within the therapeutic process in art therapy, the clients are encouraged to both create and observe the process they have gone through. One of the interviewees found it challenging to maintain high-level observation together with the student, since her sign language is not good or rich enough. Therefore, she occasionally asks the school counselor to be present in the art therapy room, with the client's approval, and they lay out the artworks in a kind of exhibition. Since the counselor's sign language is very good, they can look at the products together and raise the level of observation, thinking, and conceptualization of the works.

One of the interviewees stressed the development of the ability to use abstract concepts and that many concrete examples are often needed to illustrate an abstract notion. This can be done both verbally but also from the art world or in examples of dialogue within the artwork. For example, a concept, such as "boundaries" and "blurring boundaries", can be demonstrated very nicely using colors. In addition, she sometimes uses the writing of a key sentence or idea to hold a thought together. Similar to painting, a thought that is presented visually can be preserved in writing. For example, the art therapist can write down an interpretation and client and therapist can return to it and continue to think about it later in the session.

Working on self-portraits

One of the interviewees described work done with kindergarteners on their personal identity as D/HH children. The art therapist photographed them in black and white and let the children color their portraits. She then gave them pictures of hearing aids or the accessories that came with the implants and suggested pasting the aids to their pictures of their heads. This work can be expanded to all kinds of personal portraits and can involve observing and processing the experience as a function of the student's age and abilities. This type of work deals directly with self-identity as a D/HH student and can be implemented in different contexts as a function of the developmental process.

Working on communication with the environment

A breakdown in communication can sometimes occur during an art therapy session. In such situations like in the real world, students can be taught how to talk about misunderstandings. They can be taught how to get help from others in different contexts and the extent to which hearing and D/HH people also benefit from requests for help. One of the interviewees mentioned that she creates simulations in sessions in which the clients practice how to communicate with the environment so that they can better apply these skills to their real lives.

Group art therapy

The interviewees described ways of working with an entire small class of D/HH students and pointed to the importance of mutual influence in these groups. The ability to see what someone else is doing can expand other students' interest and ability to work with the art materials. In addition, within the group, social skills can be honed according to the age and level of functioning of the students. This can range from basic work on emotions and how to behave in a group in early childhood to more complex social skills at adolescence.

The group work begins for example by recalling the artwork that was made the previous week. During the artwork, the art therapist decides how much guidance should be given to the construction of the work. One of the art therapists felt that instructions depended on the age of the children. For example, younger children should work on separate surfaces, but older children can produce joint works. By contrast, another art therapist emphasized the importance and potential of learning from joint works from an early age since different social situations arise that can be addressed as a parallel to what happens in life outside the group (what happens when the D/HH student needs something from a friend, what happens when a friend enters the work area, how to treat a friend who is sad or frustrated, etc.). At the end of the session, the group members can observe the works together and share their experiences, which also greatly improves these students' ability to express and conceptualize. One of the interviewees who works with preschool children said that she also includes songs with lyrics at the beginning and end of the sessions.

At times, art therapists set up groups to work on certain topics. One of the interviewees described therapeutic groups that deal with sexual-social education. In her view, art in these groups can be used in diverse ways. Initially, art can help to introduce concrete concepts such as getting to know the body, naming body parts, and other topics. Later, art can be used to help students engage in abstract, more complex concepts. This can be done through structured exercises, such as asking the students to draw their idea of a beautiful woman/handsome man or drawing a line around their body and working on the body image. After the artwork, a discussion can be held on these issues and their relationship with the group members.

A number of interviewees said that they sometimes work with dyads to encourage interactions in a sufficiently limited setting that does not threaten the students. Sometimes the dyads are composed of D/HH students and the focus is both on each client's space of expression and the common space. One of the interviewees described working with pairs of students, one of whom is D/HH and the other is not. Within the art therapy room and through the art materials, each member of the dyad begins to get to know the other and make contact in a protected and safe way. At first, the artwork was more structured, but later each of the students went on to continuous personal work which revealed specific patterns of communication and the relationship between them.

In addition, parents and children can work jointly in art therapy sessions. In these groups, the goal is better acquaintance between family members. Here, too, the exercises are well defined and can include working with photos from the family album or preparing a work of art for each other. The artwork is discussed by the parent and the child and then the observation is opened up to the group. In this way, the parents also make contact and get to know each other as a support group.

An open studio

The open studio concept is a stimulating environment for older students (Heller, 2021). The open studio is a space in which students are invited to engage in free expression through art materials. Within the studio, the art therapist can have a variety of art materials available, even those that are less often used in individual work (such as woodworking). The interviewees described both the work of a class of students with D/HH and the integration of D/HH students together with students from regular classes. The possibility of integration within an open setting, where many different creative processes take place simultaneously and are mediated by an art therapist, creates an opportunity for new encounters and acquaintance with "the Other" for all participants.

Working in large formats

One interviewee emphasized the importance of working on an easel and creating in large formats. She noted that there is something compelling about large artwork that heightens self-worth and sense of visibility. Throughout the interviews, the art therapists referred to the power of art, especially in creating large and impressive projects, and their value in building students' self-confidence.

Collages

Boyle and Snow (2019) addressed ways to develop abstract thinking. In their view, working on a collage is very similar to working on sentence construction. In both cases, there are parts from which the whole can be built. In this way, the student can be helped to engage in a variety of abstract concepts that include arrangement and assembly. The interviewees also described how flipping through newspapers and selecting objects can help clients focus on their desires and preferences. This is another opportunity to expand self-identity and encounter a variety of images and objects, from which the student may be able to find something to define his/her experiences more closely.

Working with found objects

One interviewee described working with found objects (see Siano, 2016) in the art therapy room. She noted that on an emotional level, the feeling that everything has value is very significant for these students. The artwork includes connecting, gluing, and painting objects to endow them with renewed meaning. Students can work in a one-off setting or they can also work on a follow-up project over several sessions. Working with these materials often produces a feeling of success.

THE MEANING OF ART

"It gives them a gift for life", one of the interviewees told me. In her view, art strengthens D/HH students in terms of motor performance, and emotionally in that it gives them the ability to explore a variety of possibilities. The diverse experiences open up a world for them and allow them to get to know themselves in a variety of roles. Through their natural interaction with non-verbal art, they are able to communicate their experiences with the reality around them.

Another interviewee said that art is a bridge between two languages and constitutes a space for communication and connection. Art makes it possible to engage in internal processes, construct a narrative, and observe it, and invites the student on a journey with art materials. It allows for sublimation, release and venting, and diverse modes of expression. Art is designed to recognize and process emotions to better communicate them to the world.

Finally, one of the interviewees emphasized the role of artwork, in particular in the presence of a hearing art therapist. She considers that it strengthens the students' self-confidence and helps them build a bridge through art to the world of hearing people. In her view, art expands their emotional world, their modes of expression, and the feeling that others understand them.

COLLABORATIVE INTERVENTIONS INVOLVING PARENTS AND STAFF MEMBERS

Working with parents

The key differences between D/HH students are also related to the considerable differences between their parents. Most D/HH students are born to hearing parents. For many hearing parents of D/HH children, the discovery of deafness causes tensions in the parent-child relationship, leading to feelings of anxiety, inadequacy, disappointment, frustration, and guilt. The child may go through critical developmental stages without being able to communicate and discuss abstract ideas, feelings, and information about the world such as differences between reality and fantasy. As a result, these children often face challenges such as parental disconnectedness, emotional distance, difficulties in developing an identity as a person who is D/HH, and lack of exposure to deaf culture (Avrahami-Winaver et al., 2020). In addition, hearing parents often do not know how to communicate in sign language. When a student enters the education system and learns sign language, there is sometimes a gap and a breakdown in communication between these students and their parents. The interviewees all noted that in families where there are many family members with D/HH, there is a much greater acceptance, but there are also issues with respect to identifying difficulties and sometimes anger at the system, for example over a decision or recommendation to place their child in special education.

The interviewees emphasized the importance of the art therapist's relationship with the parents. This relationship can help parents view their children in a more profound way and thus be more capable of processing their difficulties, behaviors, and distress. In addition, parents can express themselves and the difficulties they are experiencing in raising a child with D/HH in a setting where they can benefit from the non-judgmental perspective, containment, and understanding on the part of the art therapist with respect to the struggles they are experiencing. The interviewees noted that the main goal is to improve the relationship between students and their parents in such a way that the parents will become an address for the students when a difficulty arises. Sometimes, the art therapist helps mediate between students and their parents. One of the complexities is deciding which staff member will be in charge of relationships with parents and in what way, so that the parents are not overwhelmed. Another issue has to do with the fact that classes for D/HH students also cater to students living further away, which complicates the parents' accessibility to the school.

One of the interviewees said that the staff invites parents of preschool children once a month to kindergarten for Parents' Day. During this meeting, the parent and child typically make a joint artwork, and the parents attend a lecture on a different topic each time of importance to them. Another interviewee who also works with preschool children said that when parents come to a joint meeting with their children in kindergarten, it is always a very meaningful experience for the children that they continue to mention.

A number of interviewees specifically addressed adolescents. In their view, the differences between chronological age, functional age, verbal age, and sexual age can be very confusing to adolescents' parents. Adolescence also increases the gap between students and their parents, especially when parents have not learned sign language. Situations arise where they feel they are less and less familiar with their child. Parental guidance can help mediate between adolescents and their parents and clarify the importance of finding a common communication channel. One interviewee described situations in which she broke the boundaries of the setting to help clients cope with the world outside the therapy room. For example, she described a client who was very afraid of taking the bus alone and her parents were also very concerned. Eventually, she decided to follow her client in her own car while the client took the bus.

Working with staff members

All the interviewees considered that working with staff members was highly important. Part of this effort involved explaining art therapy to the staff and what this field means to students. Sometimes this is done by displaying the students' artworks (with their permission) and looking at them together. This encourages staff members to observe the heterogeneity of the population and how art therapy can be used in a variety of forms and be tailored to specific students. Another alternative is to organize sessions or a workshop with staff members while working with art materials non-verbally.

One art therapist described situations where there were several classes of D/HH students within a regular school. In this type of framework, numerous very nice projects were carried such as making sign language accessible to all the students in the school and even a choir for D/HH students and hearing students who sang in sign language as well. She stressed that in these frameworks it is crucial for the staff to learn sign language. This can give students the sense that they are part of the school community and that all the community members are making an effort to interact and communicate with each other. One of the interviewees described a case in which she felt that the relationship between one of the teachers and one of the D/HH students was problematic. She decided to ask the teacher and student to work together in the art therapy room. They both agreed and began working together using art materials. This enabled the teacher to observe the student's strengths and see him in another light, which helped her build a better relationship with him.

CLINICAL ILLUSTRATION

Dana was eight years old, and in second grade, when she was referred to art therapy. She was the fifth daughter of hearing parents who worked hard for a living. She was born with a significant hearing impairment and underwent implant surgery in early childhood. Her rehabilitation was partial given her parents many other obligations. She attended a special education kindergarten for children with D/HH and learned sign language there. She started first grade in a small special education class in a regular school. In the first year, she participated in a whole-class art therapy program designed to help students process the transition experience to first grade. This year she was offered art therapy in an individual setting. Dana is small and thin, with long hair and large eyes that seem to be constantly on the lookout, and she appears scared. The teacher referred her to art therapy because she felt that Dana was lonely and frightened and had problems making contact with other students in the class and outside the class.

When the art therapist came to get Dana from the class, Dana was not sure what was expected of her. Her educator introduced her to the art therapist and told her that once a week they would meet to work together with art materials. Dana followed the art therapist with her eyes lowered, fearful of the new experience. Inside the art therapy room was a table with art materials on it. Dana immediately approached the markers and began to draw her familiar painting of sun, sky, grass, and a house. The art therapist sat down in front of Dana, in a way that Dana could see her best. She looked at Dana and smiled at her occasionally. Dana looked down. The art therapist showed her the room and told her that she could choose each week what art material to work with and what to do in the room.

The next week, Dana came to the art therapy room and sat down at the table. The art therapist sat down in front of her again. Dana chose the markers again. The art therapist smiled, which enabled Dana to relax somewhat. The art therapist indicated in sign language: "Maybe you would like to try drawing with these pencils?" Dana hesitated. Most of the time she worked with markers. Dana appeared unable to decide. The art therapist took a sheet of paper and began scribbling with the pencils. She mixed colors and created spirals in different shades. Dana seemed interested. Hesitantly she took a pencil and tried to draw with it.

The following week, Dana went back to pencils and started drawing with them. The art therapist suggested drawing together. Dana agreed. Slowly they created a drawing of the school, the many students, and also the art therapy room where Dana and the art therapist drew together. At some point, the art therapist signed that she had an idea. She brought a small jar of water and began to brush over a small part of the drawing. The pencils were water soluble and the shades began to blend with each other. Dana's eyes, which were big anyway, opened in astonishment. With a hesitant hand, she took the brush and also tried to mix the colors.

In the following weeks, Dana continued to come to the art therapy room, each time experimenting with different materials and different forms. Slowly she became acquainted with the art materials and the possibility of creating with them. At the end of each session, the art therapist would stop the creative process and they would look at the artworks together and try to summarize the process. Of all the art materials, Dana was particularly attached to acrylic paints. There was something about working with them and being able to mix colors that caught her attention.

A few months after the treatment began, the art therapist brought a large sheet of paper to the room and suggested that Dana work at the easel using acrylic paints. She suggested that Dana should paint herself. "How will I do that?" Dana asked, thus indicating that the project seemed too big for her. "You will stand, and I will draw the outline of your body and then you can paint within the contours". Dana took time to think about it. The art therapist knew that it was a challenging project, but she hoped that the many weeks Dana had already spent in the art therapy room would give her the courage to accept the new challenge. "I will help you" the art therapist added and encouraged Dana to start working together.

For two months, Dana worked on her self-portrait. In delicate lines and exciting color mixes, she painted her figure, part by part. She chose what color each item of clothing would have and how to depict the girl's long hairstyle in the painting. The art therapist sat across from her so that Dana could see her throughout the work process. Occasionally they would stop, stand in front of the painting and observe. When Dana came to draw her face, the art therapist brought a mirror and suggested she use the reflection. Dana looked and drew, imitated and drew, looked again. Slowly, two large, observing eyes emerged in the painting, this time they seemed a little less frightened to the art therapist.

SUMMARY

Art therapy for D/HH students is primarily intended to provide them with a space for communication. In the art therapy room, the language of art can be used to express a wide range of emotions and thoughts and to mediate and bridge between the different languages in the student's life. This is a non-judgmental place, where it is possible to expand the range of the students' experiences, enjoy success, and start exploring what is best for each, when, and in what way. Through concrete experiences and within art, abstract concepts can be broached, in particular their personal identity as students with D/HH.

The different languages in these students' lives sometimes challenge the therapeutic process and the art therapist needs to find a way to adapt the mode of communication to each student and be aware of the importance of observation. This includes the art therapist's observation of the clients and their body language and the clients' observation of the art therapists and their body language. Art therapists should always make sure they are positioned to have their faces visible to the client and be aware that it is often very difficult for students and sometimes impossible to create with art materials and communicate at the same time. The process is therefore often slower, so it must be given sufficient time and the space it needs. In so doing, the art therapist must also pay attention to the presence of "black holes" and make sure that what is said in the room is indeed clear and understood by the student.

The chapter described a variety of interventions in art therapy for D/HH students. The interviewees emphasized how crucial it is to expand the universe of experiences of these students in particular by exposing them to a wide range of creative materials. They recommended ongoing projects such as collages, working with found objects, or working on paintings with large formats. These projects can increase the students' confidence and self-esteem. In addition, to help them connect with their environment, they recommended a variety of ways to process their experiences in the world through simulations and constructing scenes from life using creative materials. They also recommended therapeutic sessions in pairs, groups, or in an open studio setting with D/HH students along with hearing students, to help them emerge from the bubble of loneliness and establish connections with the world around them.

REFERENCES

Avrahami-Winaver, A., Regev, D., & Reiter, S. (2020). Pictorial phenomena depicting the family climate of deaf/hard of hearing children and their hearing families. *Frontiers in Psychology*, 11. https://www.frontiersin.org/articles/10.3389/fpsyg.2020.02221/full

Boyle, H., & Snow, P. D. (2019). The value of Art therapy: An intervention to enhance emotional health of children with hearing loss. *JADARA*, 39(1), 6.

Heller, A. (2021). The "Open Studio" model in educational frameworks. In D. Regev & S. Snir, (Eds.), *Integrating art therapy into education: A collective volume.* (pp. 111–127). Routledge (Taylor & Francis Group).

Hoggard, M. (2006). Art psychotherapy with people who are deaf or hearing impaired. *International Journal of Art Therapy*, 11(1), 2–12.

Horovitz, E. G. (Ed.). (2007). *Visually speaking: Art therapy and the deaf.* Charles C Thomas Publisher.

King, N. (2020). Building a bridge between the deaf community and art therapy. *Art Therapy,* 37(2), 97–98.

Lev-Wiesel, R., & Yosipov-Kaziav, J. (2005). Deafness as reflected in self-figure drawings of deaf people. *Journal of Developmental and Physical Disabilities,* 17(2), 203–212.

Siano, J. (2016). *Holy junk: Lost, found and rejected objects in art therapy.* Self-publication.

Tapia-Fuselier, J. L., & Ray, D. C. (2019). Culturally and linguistically responsive play therapy: Adapting child-centered play therapy for deaf children. *International Journal of Play Therapy,* 28(2), 79.

BRIEF BIOGRAPHIES OF THE ART THERAPISTS WHO CONTRIBUTED TO THIS CHAPTER

Anat Avrahami-Winaver, art therapist (Ph.D.), psychotherapist, and supervisor, has worked in the education system as a kindergarten teacher for many years and for 20 years as an art therapist with adolescents with D/HH.

Einav Dimant, art therapist (M.A.), social worker, and supervisor, has worked for 15 years in the education system, including 10 years as an art therapist with adolescents with D/HH.

Einat Gebai, art therapist (M.A.), has worked as a kindergarten teacher for 13 years and for 7 years in the education system as an art therapist with adolescents with D/HH.

Yael Levin Yesod, art therapist (M.A.) and supervisor, has worked for 12 years in the education system, including 7 years as an art therapist with pre-school children with D/HH.

Tali Levkov, art therapist (M.A.) and social worker, has worked for seven years in the education system, including six years with children with D/HH.

Rula Najjar, art therapist (M.A.) and supervisor, has worked for four years in the education system as an art therapist with pre-school and elementary school children with D/HH.

Vitti Rosenzweig Kones, art therapist (M.A.) and supervisor, has worked as an art teacher for many years and for 17 years in the education system as an art therapist with students with D/HH of all ages.

Art Therapy for Blind Students or with a Severe Visual
Impairment (B/SVI)

Three

INTRODUCTION

The population of students who are blind or have a severe visual
impairment (B/SVI) is highly varied and covers students who do not
see at all and students with partial vision. In addition, visual impairment is sometimes combined with other disabilities or syndromes. In
the State of Israel, there are only a few special education frameworks
for B/SVI students, most of whom have multiple disorders. Most B/SVI
students are enrolled in the regular education system. For this reason,
it is very difficult to locate art therapists who specialize in this population. The list of interviewees at the end of the chapter is composed of
art therapists who have worked for many years with a large number of
B/SVI students, art therapists who have worked briefly with this population, and others who have only worked with a single student but felt
they had gained enough experience to be interviewed.

Art therapy with B/SVI students aims to address and is adapted to
their impaired or non-existent sense of sight. However, there is no
doubt that this impairment affects many other facets of these students'
lives. Herrmann (1995) argued that it is important to differentiate
students who were born with B/SVI from those who have memories
from the period before they lost their sight. For students who were
not born with B/SVI, there will always be a sense of lack and loss,
while for students who are born with B/SVI, this is the only condition
they have ever known, which can make it easier for them in terms of
acceptance. Other cases involve students in the process of losing their
sight or who know that they will lose their sight later in life. These
circumstances clearly affect their existence and the type of art therapy
proposed to them.

The interviewees all emphasized the tradeoff between senses. When
students cannot rely on their sense of sight, they turn to other senses.

DOI: 10.4324/9781003156918-3

This underscores the importance of helping them develop the sense of touch, hearing, and even smell. These can help them better orient themselves in space and better understand the world around them without giving up developing their sense of sight in situations where there is residual vision. One art therapist who works with young children noted that at times the development of drawing skills is slower, perhaps because of the lack of visual exposure to the drawings of others. In these cases, art materials can be used to slowly build up an understanding that artworks can represent aspects of the world around them.

Herrmann (1995) commented that in 1991 when he began to provide art therapy for B/SVI students, the general consensus was to only give these students clay that could be felt, even without sight. The possibility of letting these students paint with a variety of drawing materials was a far-fetched idea some 30 years ago. However, as discussed in this chapter, modes of intervention in art have evolved. Today most of the art therapists I interviewed work with a variety of creative materials that they adapt to each client. At the same time, most of the interviewees addressed the challenges of working with this population since art therapy focuses on the visual. The best ways to develop the field of art therapy to accommodate this population remain a complex issue, requiring creative solutions. The interviewees each described their own trajectories in tailoring interventions for these students. All consider that the effort has been rewarding and that making these art materials accessible to these students is important.

On a personal level, this was one of the more touching chapters to write. The art therapists' willingness to give their knowledge sound and meaning was very exciting. This is particularly true given the lack of literature in the field and the feeling that in different places at the same time, creative art therapists have invented different variations of the same wheel. I hope this chapter can shed some initial light on the experience I had during its writing. For me, without a doubt, this was the impetus to thinking about a field that needs to be further explored.

THE THERAPEUTIC GOALS OF ART THERAPY

McMath (2005) addressed the goals of art therapy for B/SVI children. She noted that developing B/SVI children's sense of touch, sensory awareness, and sensory experiences can contribute to their development in other important areas including mobility, spatial concepts, gross and fine motor coordination, language, body concept, Braille reading, cognitive abilities, motor skills, social relationships, emotional and conceptual acquisitions, and others. Art therapy offers B/SVI children a wide range of experiences with a variety of tactile art materials that can considerably enhance the functional use of the hands and fingers (Weiss & Rocco, 1992). Combining diverse sensory experiences complements such goals as increasing self-esteem, self-expression, communication, independence, sensory awareness, self-concept, interpersonal skills, autonomy, exploration, and self-confidence, as well as many others (McMath, 2005). Rubin (1978), an art therapist who worked with B/SVI individuals, considered that the art process provides a protective container that upholds the division between reality and fantasy. This quality gives participants the opportunity to test themselves more daringly and to openly express their fantasies (Berbrier, 2002).

The interviewees also addressed the goal of processing the difficulty and understanding the shortcomings of the students' life circumstances. Some students are born with B/SVI: this is the only state they have ever known. For this reason, it is difficult for them to understand how others perceive and experience the world around them, and what is hard for them to do as compared to the sighted. Especially for adolescents, therapeutic work centers on the construction of self-identity and the place of the disability within this developing identity.

Benjet (1993), an art therapist who also worked with B/SVI people, indicated that art not only exists as a mode of self-expression with therapeutic value, but is also a medium that enables these individuals to communicate with others who have sight (Berbrier, 2002). Since many B/SVI students are integrated into the regular education system, their daily contact with the sighted provides the basis for therapeutic work. One of the art therapists explained that a lack of visual input sometimes leads to a lack of understanding of many social situations. This points to the need for mentalization and observation of situations in which these students interact with others, both sighted or B/SVI. Another art therapist described a student with a severe visual impairment, who was clearly unaware of the existence of other students around him when he entered first grade. It was important first of all to teach him the basic social skills of acknowledging others around him. In addition, as noted by one of the art therapists, in situations where there are visual remnants, it is important to determine whether the client can recognize the faces of his/her classmates and if not, help him/her develop visual discernment skills. One possibility is to photograph the children in the class so that the client can become familiarized with their clothing, body language, etc.

All the art therapists emphasized the importance of affording these students greater independence in their lives. The core idea is that the art therapy room is a microcosm for the students' lives, and the more independently they orient themselves in the room, the greater their sense of ability and the more attempts they will make to be independent in other areas of their lives. This goal also involves working with parents. Many parents find it difficult to let their children experience independent living. Sometimes the main goal is simply to allow the students to attend treatment sessions without parental intrusion while also responding to the parents' need for guidance with respect to their child's path toward independence.

One of the art therapists drew attention to the fact that many of these students undergo numerous invasive procedures and operations. They may feel they have little control over their lives and that the world is constantly penetrating them. She described a kindergarten child who was very physically aggressive. The staff had a feeling that he was simply attacking the world that was attacking him. The primary goal for these children is to help them develop a sense of control. Through art, these students can begin to feel they are in control, first over art materials, and later over other experiences. Another art therapist stressed that because of these students' dependence on their parents, they often avoid expressing anger openly. In such cases, art therapy can help them express and vent their anger sublimatively. She described a client who took a plastic eye and stuck things in it and crushed it and then told the eye that it was broken. The art therapist looked at her and reflected the anger that had been expressed verbally and bodily. The client calmed down and asked to fix the broken eye, put glitter on it, saying that there are beautiful things in it as well. It was a groundbreaking moment in that it allowed the student to talk directly for the first time about the frustration and pain she experienced because of her visual impairment.

CHALLENGES

One of the key difficulties in working with B/SVI students is finding the right position on the continuum between dependence and independence. On the one hand, all the interviewees emphasized the importance of giving these students as much independence as possible, which can help them in their daily lives. On the other hand, in some situations, the path to independence is more complex. One art therapist mentioned a client who kept putting more and more art materials on the table, until she was unable to keep track of their locations. Sometimes she would select materials that were not suitable such as pieces of paper that were too small for her to see, thus making the process difficult to organize. Another art therapist described helping clients take their unfinished artworks off the shelf to continue working on them. He described the delicate balance between supporting, or sometimes holding the work with them to make sure they do not bump into something, and letting them to do it themselves. At times, the main focus is not the artwork but the organization that it involves, such as carrying the materials, preparing the setting, choosing the right materials, etc.

Another related concern is the amount of physical contact. The art therapists here all argued that unlike other clients, B/SVI students often need physical contact to help them get to the room, orient themselves in it, find their artwork, take it to the table, etc. The dilemma of how much physical contact is right for the client and when s/he really needs it is constantly up for discussion. Since these students rely so extensively on touch, there are times when they must be helped. This includes for example finding their artwork when it is stored with other students' works, without damaging anything.

The art therapists also mentioned independence in relation to the amount of support during the creative process. What happens when a student attempts to create something, but the therapist realizes that the end product does not at all correspond to the intent and will not be recognized by the environment? Should the student be told? How important is it that the environment recognizes and perhaps also appreciates the client's work? Does this at times come at the expense of other processes and goals? These are daily dilemmas for art therapists working with B/SVI students.

Some art therapists noted that in their experience the pace of art therapy with this population is slower and can only be accomplished in small steps. The whole process of familiarization with the art therapy room and the art materials and learning the language of art to exploit it for self-expression takes time. In addition, a great deal of mediation is required throughout, in terms of how the art materials are used, guidelines for the activity, and the interactions between group members that underpin a grasp of the social situations unfolding in the room.

One of the interviewees underscored the emotional work that art therapists themselves need to engage in. She recalled working with a young girl who gradually lost her sight. The therapist herself found it hard to process the fact that the sweet girl sitting in front of her was going blind. Another interviewee described the supervision of an art therapist whose client was about to undergo eye surgery, with a high probability that he would lose the few remnants of vision he had. She said that he was experiencing the process of becoming blind as the end of the world and she felt she had no way to help him. Within supervision, she was invited to recall her initial experience with blindness to discover what would emerge. When the art therapist was able to identify the experience of helplessness and paralysis that had arisen in her in response to the student's fears of blindness, something new was made possible in the treatment. A number of art therapists addressed their difficulty in fully understanding the experience of being with B/SVI. Some try squinting to feel what it is like to see less. Others experiment with art materials with their eyes closed to better understand what is realistic to ask clients to do and how they experience the art materials.

INTERVENTION TECHNIQUES AND DEDICATED WORKING MODELS

Adapting the art therapy room and the familiarization process

The art therapists described a variety of ways to adapt the art therapy room to this population. They all insisted on understanding each client's specific disability, and specifically what exactly the student can or cannot see. Are there any remnants of vision? Does s/he see in one area and not in another? Does s/he see colors? Is the client easily dazzled? All of these features are critical to the arrangement of the therapeutic environment. To tailor the room to each client's needs, there must be an in-depth analysis of the nature of the visual impairment.

First, the art therapy room must be accessible and have permanent places for each material. The art therapist needs to think about what must be in the room and how to arrange it in such a way that the students do not bump into objects on the floor and can reach the shelves or cabinets freely and take out art materials themselves. Some therapists described devices they invented for this purpose. For example, one art therapist asked to have a sloping work surface built for her. This way the work can be placed vertically in front of the clients, so they use the remnants of their vision to see it. Accessibility is also affected by the students' range of color vision. For example, the color of the table and whether it contrasts with the color of the paper is important. In some cases, sheets of Bristol can be inserted between the table and the work paper to increase the contrast. In addition, the art materials can be placed in colored dishes that contrast with the color of the table. For students with remnants of vision, the room must not be overly crowded with stimuli that can interfere with concentration on the artwork. One art therapist noted that she avoids bright clothing or glittery jewelry, which can distract the client.

The art therapists emphasized the importance of maintaining a limited and regular range of materials. Sometimes, it is enough to work with the basic shades of any material, since most students cannot distinguish between hues. Labels indicating color can be added in Braille, for students who read Braille. Water jars for gouache must be stable. Lighting should be strong but not dazzling. The windows need to be curtained to avoid glare. One of the interviewees stressed that she always sits at eye level, so that the students will not have to look up at her and be blinded by the light.

Students with B/SVI need time to get accustomed to art making. The art therapist should introduce him/herself and the art therapy room and allow clients to slowly learn to recognize and orient themselves independently (McMath, 2005). The interviewees stressed the importance of letting clients explore the art therapy room, including the objects in each location in the room. Completely blind students can be guided to touch the different parts of the room and what is available in each location. The locations must remain the same from session to session: there must be a designated place for games and art materials (sometimes in specific boxes or baskets to facilitate orientation).

The students should be allowed to slowly get to know the art materials in the art therapy room and the possibilities and sensations inherent to each material. They need to have the possibility to explore each material in depth. Since B/SVI students often do not see enough to learn from imitation, they need comprehensive explanations of each art material and the ways it can be used for emotional expression. Clients can be exposed to different materials with different textures (shredded paper, leaves, torn strips of newspaper, etc.) with varied scents to expand their experiences. Since their hands often act as their eyes, opportunities to touch and feel the materials can enrich their world and encourage flexibility.

One of the therapists emphasized that the layout of the room and the organization of the session should be fixed and known in advance. This is because these students have little or no control over changes in reality. In their daily lives, the room they entered yesterday may be arranged differently today. Art therapy can act successfully as an emotional container by keeping the setting of both the room and the session constant.

Developmental art therapy approaches

McMath (2005) conceptualized art therapy with B/SVI people within the framework of a developmental approach. She claimed that in the introductory sessions, the art therapist should take a more active role by helping the client decipher, identify, and explore a range of materials. As the client becomes more comfortable with the therapist, the materials, and the art process, the therapist can begin to take on the role of facilitator. The art therapist should allow the client to choose the activity or the materials to be used in the session.

Clay workshop

In the only special school for blind students in the State of Israel, there has been a clay workshop for many years. Mireille Gronner has directed it for many years, first as an art teacher and then as an art therapist. Since her background is in ceramic design, she decided to make clay the main material students encounter in art therapy. She has conducted extensive research with her students, many of whom have complex disabilities in addition to being blind, on the best ways to use clay in art therapy.

Clay is first taught technically, so that the students learn how to create a surface, a ball, how to work with engraving or embossing tools, etc. The clients are invited to move to personal expression after acquiring these basics. Sometimes, students are reluctant to touch the clay and take time to gradually adapt to it. This can be done using gloves that are removed later in the process. When the students are ready for personal expression, they are given a wooden surface with a raised rim as a framework. They can create freely, with the art therapist accompanying them and reflecting to them what she sees. When a student wants to make a particular object, a model of the specific object can be brought to the workshop to help him/her feel its shape. Note that many objects cannot be touched, so B/SVI students have no idea what they look like. For example, what does a whale look like, or the ceiling in a house? In the process of touching the model, these students get an idea of how to create the object, so that their audience can recognize it. At the end of the process, students choose whether to glaze the pieces. Some students who were sighted in the past can choose the colors they are interested in easily because the concept of color is clear to them. For students who are blind from birth, the choice of color is related to a particular object or taste. For example, green is like grass or yellow is like a lemon. This way they can decide what color they want for the glaze. The concept of color also encourages conversations about colors; for example, how colors match and how they can affect the colors of the clothes they wear to produce an aesthetic effect. The creation process ends by firing the piece into the kiln. Only successful pieces are fired; the others are recycled for further use.

Work within defined boundaries

Many art therapists have been able to find a meaningful way to work with B/SVI students each in terms of their own specializations and their favorite art materials. Most referred to working with trays with rims that provide definite boundaries; however, each used a slightly different variant. Rubin (1978) noted that raised edges, borders, or rims help B/SVI individuals identify the edges of the page and also contain their artwork.

One type of work is the use of slip (De Montmollin, 2010; Klein et al., 2020) which was adapted for B/SVI students by Mireille Gronner and researched by Miki Klein (supervised by Prof. Sharon Snir and myself), who learned this approach from her. The impetus for the use of slip with the B/SVI students came from a student's serendipitous discovery of liquid clay in a recycling bucket. Slip is a mixture of water with an additional substance that produces a thick saline-type paste. It can be made by diluting and filtering any kind of clay to make it semi-fluid. Slip work is done in general in large trays with sides, so the material can be played with in various ways without the slip dripping out. The bottom of the trays can be painted black and the slip itself can be white. This forms a contrast that also allows students with remnants of vision to see where the liquid slip is and the places where the bottom of the tray is uncovered. Slip primarily provides a sensory experience for B/SVI students and a visual experience for students with remnants of vision. Although the main thrust of the activity is the experience and not the product, the design can be preserved on black or dark paper so that the white slip will stand out. Glue can be sprayed on top to keep the dried slip in place.

Another art therapist described working with paint inside trays. Liquid paints, glue, and three-dimensional materials such as small beads can be poured into the trays for the students to play with. This provides the students with a sense of control since they decide what to put in the tray and the flow of the colors and materials by moving their hands. In addition, students can decide whether to insert into the work intermediary tools such as a brush or stick or work with their fingers. Paper can be placed at the bottom of the tray so that a product remains at the end of the work.

Another alternative is to work with shaving foam inside a tray. It can be combined with finger paints and 3D materials like beads. The shaving foam activity allows for flatwork and slightly higher constructions. At the end, the work can be imprinted on paper and preserved to make a permanent artwork.

Learning general concepts in the art therapy room

Since B/SVI students often have problems understanding concepts that they are unable to see or feel at all, such as what a house looks like, a roof, a ceiling, and scale models can be made in art therapy. For example, students can make models of their home or their favorite playground. This gives these students a better sense of proportion and navigation. Art therapy work can help experience the environment in a way that does not embarrass clients.

Complex concepts can also include abstract or physical notions. One art therapist described a student who had difficulty understanding how to make a circular motion. She took him to the potter's wheels and put his hands on the wheels as they turned. Once his body sensed the rotational motion, he learned to do it in a variety of contexts including creating a ball of clay and mixing a salad in a bowl.

The no-fail method of painting and drawing (Benjet, 1993)

This method was reported in the literature three decades ago (Benjet, 1993). The art therapist or client coats the entire surface of the canvas or paper with paint or glaze to provide an overall background of color and depth. The art therapist then applies pieces of quarter-inch black masking tape to the canvas or paper to delineate key regions of the picture in process. The therapist then asks the client what images he or she would like to place in each area (for example within the sky area). If the client does not express any preferences, the therapist can make suggestions. The therapist addresses one area of the picture and one image at a time to make the process accessible to the client. Once the client has decided on an image, the therapist or client then creates its outline in masking tape on the canvas or paper. The client is encouraged to select a color for the image and to paint within the tape outline. The client then paints around all the images. All the masking tape is then removed, leaving outlines in the color of the underpainting to provide contrast with the newly applied paint. If the client prefers, the tape may be left as part of the finished work. The interviewees also described the use of adhesive paper and stickers of various types to help even completely blind students to paint. The stickers can be used to represent all kinds of images. The students can use touch to locate the stickers and work with color between them.

Group art therapy

A number of interviewees described the value of group work with B/SVI students. In Israel, this work takes place mainly in two main frameworks. The first is in the special education school for B/SVI students. The second is a framework for students who are enrolled in different schools but who meet together for group work in the afternoon. These groups deliberately associate students with similar characteristics. The purpose of these programs is to promote communication and forge ties between these students, which is part of its appeal.

The art therapists who led these groups all emphasized that the setting is crucial. The students need to know in advance where to sit and what to do during each phase of the session. At the start, the art therapist explains what materials are on the table and how they can be used. One of the art therapists said that she presents the art materials individually to each client, after a great deal of thinking about what materials are suitable and how to present them in containers that will help the students orient themselves. When these groups also include blind students and not just students with visual impairments, art materials that can be fingered and are primarily in 3D are prioritized. Students are given art materials individually and work on their own artwork. The work is usually centered on a specific theme, such as the construction of each participant's personal story using creative materials. Sometimes students work together in pairs, or even the whole group can work on one surface to combine the individual products into a joint artwork. In other cases, the interactions are mostly verbal. At the end of the session, the students are invited to share their artwork. Sometimes a specific or alternating song closes the session.

One of the therapists described a very successful B/SVI photography group assisted by a photographer. At first, she wondered whether and how photography with this population could be used at all. Clients with visual remnants observed and chose what to photograph. For the completely blind students, the situation was more challenging. The solution was that they went outside with the arts therapist who described what she saw and let them feel the environment as much as possible. They stopped her whenever there was something in the description, sound, or smell that caught their attention and then a picture was taken. When the photographs were developed, the therapist explained what was seen in each frame, which was then transcribed. This generated a great deal of excitement and an experience of success. The program ended with an exhibition attended by family members and friends.

Another art therapist described groups she leads in a regular school, where she integrates B/SVI students with sighted students from their class. She described a specific student with a severe visual impairment who had little perception of his surroundings. She paired the client with a strong student, who walked him to the art therapy room and responded to his artwork. Later, they also started playing together and forged a bond.

Verbal interventions

The interviewees described two types of verbal interventions specific to this population. The goal of the first verbal intervention is to clarify the experience of vision. Because these students do not see, they sometimes miss important information. For example, the therapist needs to explain how to do each activity or how the art materials can be used. Sometimes they also fail to capture social information. For example, if someone stumbles and drops something in their vicinity, these students may misconstrue it as an aggressive gesture. Similarly, B/SVI students may not parse expressions of anger between students correctly. All of these situations require verbal mediation. The second type of verbal intervention is aimed at palliating a lack of full vision. One of the art therapists described a conversation with a client who was working in a tray with shaving foam and finger paints. Suddenly, a beautiful rainbow of colors emerged. The art therapist responded with admiration but had to explain the disparity between what she saw and the girl's tactile experience.

THE MEANING OF ART

Many of the art therapists stated that art helps these students express themselves and shows them that they are capable of engaging in activities just like other students. The difficulties that arise in the creative process can also occur in daily life. The possibilities and solutions provided through work with the art materials can lead to discussions about possibilities and solutions in the real world as well. One of the art therapists described discovering in art therapy groups that certain B/SVI children are very, very talented. They themselves were not aware of it. This gave them a great deal of empowerment when classmates and teachers admired their products. In fact, art provided them with a new additional pathway to excellence and success and constituted a bridge to helping them find their place in society. Finally, some therapists addressed the sense of calm that art materials impart to students. Because the hands are such a significant organ, contact with the material often becomes relaxing, especially when they can choose the material they prefer to use for artwork.

COLLABORATIVE INTERVENTIONS INVOLVING PARENTS AND STAFF MEMBERS

Working with parents

All the art therapists emphasized that working with parents varies considerably as these children grow up. When the children are very young, part of the work involves helping parents deal with the fact that they have a child with B/SVI, a child who is gradually losing his/her vision or a child born with some syndrome who must deal with a wide range of medical problems. Accompaniment in these stages of grief processing is crucial and requires containment on the part of the treatment staff. In addition, many children undergo numerous medical examinations, including invasive procedures, where family accompaniment can be determinant. Older students face additional challenges, as the degree of independence required of them by society increases. Art therapists can accompany parents through all these stages, by trying to find the right balance for them and their child between guarding and protecting and independence.

The special school for B/SVI students organizes an end-of-the-year exhibit of artworks made in art therapy. Students can choose whether they want to display their artworks or not. Other students from the school are invited and can touch the works on display. Parents, friends, and staff admire the students' creations. However, it forces art therapists to think about finding the ways for the works to be understood by others to grasp what the student intended.

Joint workshops for parents and students can also be organized. For example, one of the art therapists suggested working on shared surfaces where the parent and child choose how to represent their hands and where to position them. While working with clay, they can choose whether to emboss or engrave. Another art therapist suggested holding special sessions for parents and children together during the holiday season where one of the holiday symbols can be produced together (e.g., a Hanukkah menorah).

The Ministry of Education of the State of Israel operates 12 centers that cater to the B/SVI and provide support services to these students in their area. A district supervisor is responsible for the work of support teachers, who coordinate the support system for these students in the educational frameworks. Recognizing that B/SVI affects not only vision, but has wider implications for student functioning, the National Supervision for Students with Sensory Impairments established a national multidisciplinary team who specializes in this field. It is composed of an occupational therapist, a speech therapist, a physiotherapist and is currently led by an arts therapist, Shelly Meroz. This team provides training primarily to support teachers who then transfer what they learn to the educational and therapeutic teams that work with these students in the educational settings. Support teachers can turn to this specialized team for supervision when problems arise with a specific student. Prior to the supervision session, the support teacher fills out a questionnaire that provides broad functional data on the student. The supervision session is attended by the educational and therapeutic staff (which may include an educator/kindergarten teacher, counselor, integration teacher, and arts therapist, if any), who work with the student in the educational framework. On the day of the supervision session, the external multidisciplinary team is convened for a joint supervision session with the local staff working with the student. Each member of the team presents questions and specific recommendations. This leads to brainstorming to better respond to the student in an integrative way. For example, when the local staff raises difficulties about a student's difficulty in maintaining personal space (a seemingly simple concept for a sighted student but very abstract for a student with B/SVI), the multidisciplinary team can offer intervention tools such as clarifying the concept by illustrating it via the body or going to the playground to experience a personal space on the equipment, demonstrating the usual distance concretely, or reading stories that deal with the subject. One of the questions that often arise in these sessions is: "What is blindness to you?" This type of introspection contributes to a better understanding of attitudes and approaches to working with these students. At the end of the session, the multidisciplinary team provides written recommendations and insights for further work with the student, which are implemented in full collaboration with the support teacher and the local staff and are tailored to the nature of the framework. Some of the recommendations may also include work on emotions in arts therapy. If necessary, a follow-up session on the student is scheduled.

One art therapist described how important it is for staff members to put themselves in the students' shoes. This can be done by putting on glasses with different corrections. These "training glasses" mimic vision problems in which part of the field of vision is blocked (damage to the central or peripheral vision), vision problems where the color spectrum is reduced to shades of grey, problems with glare, and others.

CLINICAL ILLUSTRATION

Six-and-a-half-year-old Ido lost his sight in a car accident when he was five. In his final year in kindergarten and after a long hospitalization, he took his first steps in the world of the blind. This transition was not easy for him and his family saw him turn inward. When he entered first grade, the situation deteriorated further. Although it was clear to all around him that he was capable of learning like all children, the transition to a new framework was traumatic. He would come to class in the morning and sit in the same chair until the end of the day. Attempts by his friends and staff to take him out into the yard or move around the classroom were met with outright refusal. The support teacher also tried to help, but until Ido's emotional state had been addressed, it appeared that it would be impossible to address other facets of his life.

The multi-professional staff were unsure how to encourage Ido to go to the art therapy room. On the one hand, it was clear he needed help. On the other hand, it was also clear that it would be difficult to take him to the therapy room and it was even clearer that he would certainly not go alone. After much deliberation, it was decided to recruit his classmate Hila to come with him to art therapy in a dyadic setting. Hila, whose parents had divorced the previous summer, also needed emotional support, but she seemed attentive and sensitive enough to help Ido.

The first week the art therapist came to class. She sat down next to Ido and started talking to him. She brought a lump of modeling clay with her and put it in his hand. Hesitantly Ido began to knead the modeling clay and together they tried to spread it on a pre-prepared surface. Ido was distant but did not refuse the joint work. The modeling clay seemed to remind him of his kindergarten days and something in him calmed down. The art therapist told him that next week he would go with Hila once a week to the art therapy room. She assured him that the room was close by, that it had a lot of art materials, and that Hila would help him go back and forth. Ido hesitated and said he would think about it. The art therapist saw the dilemma in his eyes.

A week later when Ido came to the school, Hila was already waiting for him at the gate. She helped him put his bag in the classroom and reminded him that today they had their first session of art therapy. Ido had known Hila since kindergarten. Although he hesitated, Hila put her little hand in his and led him to the art therapy room. The art therapist was waiting for them at the door and Ido could not help but be fascinated by Hila's endless chatter and the pleasant atmosphere in the therapy room.

The following weeks were spent getting to know the art therapy room. Hila emerged as a patient and attentive teacher. She walked around the room with Ido and introduced him to a different corner in the art therapy room each time. Slowly, slowly Ido began to move independently, groping with his hands and exploring his surroundings. The art therapist cleared space in the room and made sure that the art materials were in permanent places. Ido remembered that he once loved to paint but was sure he could not do it again. At first, he only agreed to work with modeling clay or wet clay, which are materials that can be felt and shaped in a certain way. It was very important to him that Hila understand what he had created, and he would consult with her from time to time to make sure that what he was doing was indeed understood by her.

At the same time, Hila began to lead Ido during the classroom breaks as well. He slowly agreed to move around the school and with the help of the support teacher he also learned to navigate. His parents were asked to come in for parental guidance and began to digest the dramatic change that had taken place in their lives. Ido's progress moved them and the art therapist, with Ido's consent, showed them some of the artworks he had begun to make in art therapy.

After a few months, the art therapist asked Ido if he wanted to paint. "How can I?" Ido asked. "I do not see anything". The art therapist brought Ido and Hila a joint tray with a rim. She placed a sheet of paper in the bottom of the tray. She handed them gouache paints and told Ido what color was in each container. She suggested that they pour colors on the paper and use a brush to apply the paint. Ido and Hila started working together. It was the first time they had worked on a joint substrate. Hila described everything that emerged on the page to Ido. Together they decided how to move the colors and what to add to their painting. The excitement was enormous. Hila was very enthusiastic about the colors mixing together and her excitement spread to Ido as well. At the end of the session, they asked the art therapist to show the painting to their educator. The art therapist hesitated a bit but understood the value of the request. They invited the educator during the break to the art therapy room and the wide smile spread across the children's faces made it clear that a new path had indeed been created.

SUMMARY

There are several main goals in art therapy with B/SVI students. Since one of the main senses is impaired, it is crucial to help them develop the other senses. A variety of experiences in the art therapy room that activate the sense of touch, the remnants of the sense of sight if any, and also sometimes the sense of smell, can help them develop these senses. In doing so and while getting acquainted with the variety of art materials, students can begin to express their personal experiences. These experiences also include processing the difficulties they are facing and the role of the disability in their lives. All of the art therapists interviewed addressed the goal of independence and emphasized that their aim is to allow students to be as independent as possible in the art therapy room. This experience can increase their sense of control and capability in their daily lives.

Independence in the art therapy room was also emphasized as the main challenge in treatment. Art therapists described the difficulty of finding the right place on the continuum between independence and dependence and adapting their stance as a function of the client's evolving condition. The amount of physical contact with the client and the amount of support s/he receives during the work is an out-growth of the degree of independence. This issue requires a great deal of thought and supervision, since it is likely that the degree of independence that an art therapist allows students also depends on countertransference and what the concepts blindness, dependence, and independence mean to him/her. Another challenge that emerged is the pace of treatment, which is relatively slow because the students' art materials need to be accessible, and they must be helped to iden-tify the possibilities inherent to them. Many therapists also addressed their difficulties in understanding the experience of B/SVI and their attempts to place themselves in similar settings.

The art therapists described a variety of interventions for these students. They emphasized the importance of adapting the art therapy room to this population and giving the students sufficient time to get to know it. This is especially complex when the students are in different schools and the art therapist works with one or more B/SVI students in a clinic that is also adapted to other students. In order to help them acquire independence, a developmental approach sensitive to the changing demands of dependence and independence is needed. The clay workshop is highly appropriate for students who are com-pletely blind. Working within defined boundaries or using adhesives and stickers can help these students experiment with painting as well. Art therapy can help impart concepts that are sometimes difficult for these students to represent by creating scale models. Group art therapy enables students to interact socially and share experiences. This frame-work of the afternoon meetings for students with B/SVI enrolled in regular settings in different localities emerged as important and sig-nificant. Finally, the art therapists also emphasized the importance of verbal interventions while working, which helps these clients clarify the experience, understand how to use materials, and mentalize the experience where the therapist sees something which they perceive in another modality.

REFERENCES

Benjet, R. (1993). The no-fail method of painting and drawing for people who are blind or visually impaired. *American Journal of Art Therapy*, 32(1), 22–25.

Berbrier, J. (2002). *Mental imagery and dreams: art therapy with visually impaired adolescents* (Doctoral dissertation, Concordia University).

De Montmollin, D. (2010). *The barbotine game-challenge of creativity*. Editions la Revue de la ceramique et du verre. Decker Snoeck.

Herrmann, U. (1995). A Trojan horse of clay: Art therapy in a residential school for the blind. *The Arts in Psychotherapy, 22*(3), 229–234.

Klein, M., Regev, D., & Snir, S. (2020). Using the clay Slip Game in art therapy: A sensory intervention. *International Journal of Art Therapy, 25*(2), 64–75.

McMath, S. (2005). *An art therapy approach: Children who are blind and hypersensitive to touch* (Doctoral dissertation, Concordia University).

Rubin, J. (1978). *Child art therapy: Understanding and helping children grow through art*. Van Nostrand Reinhold.

Weiss, R., & Rocco, G. (1992). Art therapy. In E. Trief (Ed.), *Working with visually impaired young students: A curriculum guide for birth-3 year olds*. (pp. 117–133). Charles C Thomas Pub Limited.

BRIEF BIOGRAPHIES OF THE ART THERAPISTS WHO CONTRIBUTED TO THIS CHAPTER

Tehila Cahana, art therapist (M.A.), has worked as an art teacher for six years and currently for five years in the education system as an art therapist. For the last two years, she has worked with children with severe visual impairments or blindness in a special education kindergarten.

Tzipi Ekstain, art therapist (M.A.), has worked for 20 years as a teacher and another 12 years as an art therapist in the education system. She has worked for six years as an art therapist for students with severe visual impairment or blindness.

Mireille Gronner, art therapist and supervisor, has worked as an art teacher in a special education school for students with severe visual impairments or blindness for 15 years and as an art therapist in the same school for another 14 years.

Hiam Khaskia, art therapist (M.A.) and supervisor, has worked for 17 years as an art therapist in the education system. Over the last few years, she has worked with an adolescent with a visual impairment.

Miki Klein, art therapist (M.A.), has worked for one year in a special education school for students with severe visual impairments or blindness.

Shelly Meroz, dance and movement therapist (M.A.) and supervisor, has worked for 21 years in the education system. In the last nine years she has served as a supervisor in a multi-disciplinary team for arts therapists and staff members working with students with severe visual impairment or blindness.

Meytal Sela, art therapist (M.A.), has worked for 14 years as a teacher in the education system with students with cortical visual impairments or blindness. For the last four years she has worked as an art therapist in the education system. She worked for two years as an art therapist with a group of students with severe visual impairments or blindness.

Yehudith Tal (Tuaf), art therapist (M.A.) and supervisor, has worked as an art teacher in the education system for 10 years and for the last 20 years as an art therapist. She has worked for a few years with students with severe visual impairments or blindness.

Four

INTRODUCTION

Autism spectrum disorder (ASD) is a lifelong condition that presents on a continuum from high to low functioning (Van Lith et al., 2017). The characteristics of children with ASD vary, but some of its defining features include a tendency to withdraw from social contact, specific forms of information processing, repetitive and obsessive behaviors, and an increased sensitivity to crowds and to stimuli in general such as sounds, smells, and tactile materials (Epp, 2008; Schweizer et al., 2014).

All the art therapists interviewed for this chapter emphasized that each individual child diagnosed with ASD is different and that it would be very difficult to generalize from client to client. As noted by Dr. Stephen Shore: "If you've met one person with autism, you've met one person with autism". These differences are not only related to age and level of functioning but also to the specific ways in which ASD is expressed in each person. Even at the level of communication, there are considerable differences between verbal students and those who have little language (and sometimes communicate through alternative supportive forms), as well as the specific ways communication takes place. For example, in students who have echolalia, it is sometimes hard for others to determine what content is related to their authentic expression and what is related to repetition.

One out of five art therapists in the Netherlands and one out of six art therapists in the US treat clients with autism. Children with autism are often referred to art therapy for problems with self-image, self-expression, flexibility, and social and learning problems (Schweizer et al., 2019). Communication with the art therapist is described as a safe place to stimulate change (Schweizer et al., 2014). When discussing her own lived experience, the prominent autistic researcher Temple

DOI: 10.4324/9781003156918-4

Grandin argued that art therapy can address sensory issues that are generally associated with ASD. Her work highlights how people who have ASD tend to "think in pictures", the title of her autobiography was published in 1995 and updated in 2008 (*Thinking in Pictures, Expanded Edition: My Life with Autism*).

The art therapists interviewed here described making contact and gaining the client's confidence through treatment that is often slower, unfolds at a slower pace, and is frequently tailored to meet each client's needs. This is mainly due to these students' fear of the unfamiliar, but also the need on the part of the art therapist to invest time and thought into the best ways to present and use the creative materials available in the art therapy room and the possibilities inherent to them. One of the interviewees suggested that these clients' sense of play space is impaired, such that the issue of what is concrete and what is symbolic permeates both art and dialogue.

THE THERAPEUTIC GOALS OF ART THERAPY

The main goal when working with students with ASD is to develop communication and connection with the other. In this respect, art is considered another language that can both foster self-expression and serve as a bridge to verbal expression. A survey conducted by Van Lith et al. (2017) reported that the prime goal of most art therapists was developing social skills. One art therapist interviewed for this chapter nevertheless insisted that despite the vital importance of communication and connection with the other, it is equally crucial to help these students develop their self and true desires and rely less on others. Contact with the other and the way to engage without being dependent emerged as a core therapeutic endeavor with these students.

Another equally important goal defined by Van Lith et al. (2017) is behavior regulation. One art therapist interviewed for this chapter who works with middle- and lower-functioning students stated that in the school where she works, she observed instances of self-harm but also cases where students hurt others, primarily out of anxiety. She considers that one important goal in art therapy is relaxation, although finding a way to regulate each student requires a great deal of observation and attunement.

Schweizer et al. (2014) addressed the rigidity that may sometimes manifest when starting to work with children with ASD in art therapy. This is characterized by difficulties in flexibility and exploration and can be observed through the specific contact with the art materials and the repeated images produced during the creative work. Attempting to address these issues within treatment can clearly become a therapeutic goal. One interviewee indicated that certain art therapists, especially at the beginning of their careers, may respond to these students' rigidity by a rigid approach on their part. In her view, the opposite approach consisting of interacting flexibly and gently with the client should be used. In addition, contact with the art materials can expand the range of possibilities and may serve to address the sensory regulation problems that are present in some ASD students through experience with different forms of contact and textures. One of the art therapists also described how she works to expand the verbal communication within the therapeutic session by devoting a specific time to conversing with the student about personal experiences or reactions to the artwork. In her experience, this approach enhances the students' ability to share and tell.

Although an apparent lack of imagination and abstract thinking skills constitute one of the three major deficits of autism, paradoxically it is the one the least often addressed by most art therapists (Martin, 2009). One of the art therapists noted that a key goal is to develop the students' sense of symbolic space in terms of the ability to play and create with art materials and in terms of the discourse after the artwork.

Another goal is to develop the emotional space. One of the interviewees considered that in many cases, conceptualization in terms of knowing, acknowledging, and expressing feelings has not emerged in these students. Emotion, for the child with ASD, is identified, at best, as a bodily sensory sensation rather than an emotion. Since emotion is not expressed, the therapist often does not understand and is in what Bion termed a "place of unknowing" (1994). The therapist needs to parse the experience and then identify and conceptualize the emotion for the student. According to her, the shared experience can produce something new that is more helpful to the student than interpretation. Bion suggested metaphorically that each of these students has a soul that wants to meet the other, and for that to happen, the therapist must sometimes be willing to be in a position of unknowing, to relinquish the need to organize, to demand, to understand.

Schweizer et al. (2014) discussed the goal of raising these students' self-esteem. This goal pertains to a greater extent to high-functioning and older students, who can better perceive their environment and identify the differences between them and other students. One of the art therapists described a client with high-functioning ASD who asked numerous questions about his autism. He primarily wanted to know why he "deserved" having ASD. In the art therapy room, the goal was to observe his evolving identity as a person with ASD and to promote self-advocacy, which involves recognizing ASD and its meaning.

Another issue that emerged as a specific goal within the education system has to do with the transitions between frameworks. Because these students find it difficult to cope with changes in their lives, any such change requires a great deal of preparation, accompaniment, and thinking. For example, art therapists who work with first graders help these students adjust to the new school system. Therapists help graduating students review and recapitulate their school years and prepare emotionally for the transition to after-school life (employment, life in a hostel, or other settings).

CHALLENGES

The interviewees emphasized the key challenge of finding the best channel of communication for each client. In their view, each student with ASD represents a whole world that needs to be understood and treated on its own. Thus, what can be learned from interactions with one client may not transfer or be applicable to another. Individual students' skills, abilities, and difficulties require careful observation to develop appropriate interventions. One interviewee who works with middle- and lower-functioning students stated that she constantly challenges herself to better define the meaning of art therapy for her clients. What is actually going on inside them during the treatment? What concerns them and what does not? In what way is art therapy meaningful to them?

Creating a strong therapeutic alliance is essential to the therapeutic process. This is a paradox, given the difficulty of students with ASD to form bonds (Evans & Dubowski, 2001). One interviewee described her cautious maneuvering between wanting to draw students out of their bubble and understanding their needs, in particular within the education system where they are constantly called upon to communicate. She stressed the benefits of the protective space of the art therapy room where these pressures do not exist, although remaining in the autistic bubble impinges on the relationship and therapeutic alliance. The same therapist also stated that it is not always clear to her the extent to which she is a subject for the client and not just an object.

The need for order and organization and the difficulty making changes and transitions for these students can make the structuring of a therapeutic setting very difficult, especially in a school environment, where there are ongoing changes and constraints. Even within the art therapy room, dealing with this topic is not easy for art therapists. The art therapists interviewed here talked about how students obsessively arrange the art materials according to color or symbol, week after week. One of the therapists described a student with high-functioning ASD who talked abundantly about his developing identity as a person with ASD. At the same time, there was repetition in the content which came up in each session, thus making it difficult to understand whether the processing in previous sessions had an impact.

Osborne (2003) cautioned that art therapists should be cognizant of behavioral problems in ASD students and avoid taking a didactic position at the expense of the therapeutic stance. These behaviors can include outbursts of rage, which can lead to physical harm to themselves or others, especially in response to outside pressures. Within the education system, art therapists cannot help but be aware of such situations that also occur outside the art therapy room. Many art therapists expressed frustration that this penetrates the art therapy room and threatens the integrity of the therapeutic bubble. Inappropriate behavior can also lead to clashes with the staff, especially when the art therapist has a more containing and gentler approach.

Many art therapists noted that they often feel that they do not exist or do not interest the client. Sometimes students seem disconnected and immersed in themselves. In other cases, this can be expressed in endless details, sometimes without providing any indication that they have heard or understood what is being said. There are times when it manifests in endless questions, sometimes about things the art therapists are not qualified to answer. Feeling superfluous poses challenges to therapists. They may find that telling the student something about themselves apparently does not appear to affect or interest them at all. Lower functioning students tend to exhibit a greater lack of interest. One art therapist went so far as to use the word "emptiness" to describe her feelings. The same art therapist also described a situation where a client painted over everything he and the therapist had done together, thus "erasing" her. Alvarez et al. (1999) argued that the therapist should not ignore these feelings but rather should engage in intensive interaction with the client, even when not much seems to be happening, despite causing the therapist boredom, anxiety, or despair. One interviewee suggested having the attitude that every client has a healthy side, a part of the mind that wants communication and connection. It is precisely this side that she is looking for and wants to make contact with in art therapy.

INTERVENTION TECHNIQUES AND DEDICATED WORKING MODELS

Ways to deal with difficulties in sensory regulation

Many students living with ASD are hyper- or hypo-sensitive to touch. Some art materials may be over-stimulating as a result of tactile hypersensitivity, such as modeling materials and various types of clay. Pre-art activities such as indirect exploration of the material are often helpful. For example, placing clay in a plastic Zip-lock bag allows the student to touch it through the buffer of the bag. This allows for exploration of the fundamental properties of the material without actual direct access (Alter-Muri, 2017). When a student with ASD is excited, frustrated, or not engaged, the art therapist can recommend the use of mandala drawings to act as a centering, soothing device (Gazeas, 2012).

The art therapists interviewed here noted the importance of paying attention to the specific regulatory aspects of each student. Sometimes even presenting the art materials in a different way or reducing stimuli in the room or on the table can help the student enter into the creative process better. One of the interviewees described a student who would make himself gouache and had to put in all the colors every time. First, he would press the tube of paint all the way and it would be difficult for him to regulate the amount of pressure and the amount of paint. Over time, with the mediation of the art therapist, he learned to squeeze the right amount of paint. Another therapist described a student working with nail polish. This student needed strong smells, so she brought bottles to work. The art therapist thought that the smell of nail polish made the student feel at home.

One of the art therapists suggested that the non-crystallized areas in clients should be responded to by non-crystallized creative materials. For example, she provides finger paints in small bowls, each with its own spoon. The intended association is something primary and perhaps related to feeding. Each student is given a piece of cardboard to work on. A towel is placed underneath the cardboard that can absorb the excess liquid. Slowly, in later therapeutic sessions, sand, water, a dropper, or other materials can be provided. This type of artwork is very sensory, and the product is less important than the art making. In her opinion, the role of the art therapist is to contain the work that takes place in the room, whether liquids in containers or small pieces of paper in boxes or bowls. Once students are able to organize their work with primary materials, they can move on to materials that result in a product such as gouache or dough. In other words, the transition corresponds to a gradual developmental progression. One example of a developmental transition within this type of artwork is the recognition of the other. For example, one client drowned small dolls in a mass of paint and water. The therapist took one doll and said it was hers and should not be drowned. In so doing, she drew attention to the boundary between what was his and under his control and what was someone else's.

Dealing with repetitiveness

To help clients stay regulated and need less repetitiveness and rituals that occur in conjunction with anxiety, some interviewees stated that they make sure to maintain the same setting from session to session and keep regular hours. This way the art therapy room stays tidy, and the students actually know what to expect from session to session. Some art therapists also plan the order of activities in the session to help regulate anxiety. At the same time, one of the art therapists emphasized the importance of also accepting repetitiveness.

Alter-Muri (2017) described the case of a student who wanted to repeatedly draw the number nine. She showed him works of art that contained numbers. Slowly he began to focus more on the background for the numbers than on the digits themselves. The validation of the possibility of starting an artwork by drawing a number allowed him to expand his expression. One of the art therapists stressed the importance of introducing clients to the works of art of well-known artists as a way of giving meaning to their works, while looking for the common features. A number of art therapists talked about the importance of embarking on a creative journey from a starting point that interests the student. If, for example, the student is interested in airplanes and is willing to draw the same airplane every week, the starting point will be to expand the way the airplane is presented and later perhaps to produce more airplanes, to enrich the expression while maintaining the client's motivation to create. One interviewee noted that sometimes in order to expand the possibilities of creation, she will also intervene in the way the client works; for example, by suggesting a wider brush, working at the easel, using a different size page or switching from two-dimensional to three-dimensional images.

One interviewee described a case where at the beginning of the treatment the student took her hand, told her exactly what to draw and how, and corrected her when it was inaccurate. She felt that the use of her hand gave the student reassurance. Over time he continued to work with characters, but they were given names and emotions could be associated with them. He showed her his world in his own way and at his own pace.

Combining the artwork with other modalities (play, movement)

One art therapist described how students' symbolic play can be expanded through art making. She begins by attempting to understand the meaning of a particular type of play for the student and only then suggests expansions. For example, one student played with cars repeatedly. She suggested making a garage for the car, a place that would be the child's private space. The content came from the student and the therapist provided the art materials that expanded the experience.

Another art therapist said that she intentionally works in a large art therapy room so that students can wander around during sessions. She indicated that when she worked in a smaller room, she had the impression that some students felt they were trapped. She described a client who occasionally walks around the room and then comes back. She feels that this helps her to regulate. Other art therapists stressed that the range of options should be very wide, go beyond the art materials, and include musical instruments, dolls, hoops, or other equipment the therapist considers useful.

Using drawing as a tool for development

Martin (2008) discussed ways in which drawing can serve as a tool for student development. The first is to promote the developmental stages of drawing. As students acquire more advanced techniques, for example moving from scribble to pre-schematic and schematic drawings, their ability to express themselves develops. In addition, portraiture, for example, can be used with teenagers. Observing the model while drawing may encourage observing changes in emotional states as well.

Using comics or other creative ways to tell the client's story

The art therapist can ask students (usually high functioning ones) to draw a comic strip. This kind of artwork can become an avenue of expression for children with practical language skill difficulties. They can invest intellectually and emotionally while integrating their personal experiences as they view and reflect on their own creative work. The art therapist can also gain insights into what the student is experiencing, which is not readily available through verbal channels (Epp, 2008).

Another project that can be incorporated into art therapy to work on socialization problems is an applied behavioral technique called the Social Story (Gazeas, 2012). "Social stories are brief structured stories that describe specific social situations that one might encounter and appropriate responses to the social stimuli that will be encountered in that situation" (Scheuermann & Webber, 2002, p. 214).

For example, Kieran displays disruptive behavior getting on and off his school bus... Kieran's target social situation is getting on the bus. Social stimuli that Kieran will encounter in this situation include lining up with peers, getting his backpack and coat on, and sitting on the bus keeping hands and feet to himself. The goal will be for Kieran to read his social story before getting on the bus. The social story consists of 2 to 5 sentences and is written from the reader's perspective. Three types of sentences are included: 1) Descriptive sentences provide information about the social context; 2) Directive sentences tell the student what to do; 3) Perspective sentences describe feelings of individuals involved in the situation.

(Gazeas, 2012)

Visual diaries

One art therapist described her work with visual diaries. The art therapist and the student choose the format in terms of how many pages it will have, what size it will be, and what types of pages it will contain (in different colors, in different textures). They sew the diary pages together and work on a double page from the diary during each session. The student can work with a combination of creative techniques, including cutting and pasting. The diary establishes a regular procedure for the sessions, which can lower anxiety levels. Within the defined and maintained setting, work can proceed relatively freely. Everything can be changed in the diary and the same page can be used over and over again. Written passages produced by the student or dictated to the art therapist can also be included. The entire therapeutic process is documented within the diary, which helps to maintain continuity and makes it possible to go back and forth in time. Diaries are also appropriate in a group setting where the work can be individualized, or only involve a certain technique or certain materials or even content presented by the therapist such as a song or theme. During the Covid-19 lockdowns, students took their diaries home and met via Zoom or face to face and continued working together. At the end of the year, a closing ceremony can be held through the diary which can consist of a joint drawing or writing to each other or include a request from a significant person to write something to them in the diary. The diary helps bring closure to the treatment.

Joint drawings

In a study I conducted with Prof. Sharon Snir from Tel Hai College on the contribution of art materials to working with children with ASD (Regev & Snir, 2013), some of the art therapists raised important issues about the use of joint drawings with ASD children. They noted that working jointly on a single page brings together the two art makers in a situation in which they have to relate to each other, and thus encourages interpersonal interaction. The shared space can also provide an opportunity for modeling, where the art therapist creates something and invites the client to expand his or her repertoire of graphic expression. However, some of the interviewees described situations with this technique in which the client was wary of any intimacy, and the need for separateness made it impossible to work together on a single sheet of paper. The interviewees resolved this by seeking to establish cooperation using reciprocal attentiveness and observation, but with two separate sheets of paper. In this manner, each art maker could manifest his or her attentiveness to the other on the page, yet without the threat of intimate sharing and within the protected limits afforded by the separate spaces.

The widespread use of joint drawings with this population takes on different forms with different art therapists. Sometimes the joint drawing is open and allows for dialogue whereas in others the art therapist presents a range of specific interventions to make contact with the student (e.g., a joint squiggle). One art therapist noted that during these joint drawings, the students learn to adapt and create a coherent drawing. Another art therapist talked about a student who needed the therapist to draw alongside her and could not engage in the creative process or persevere in any other setting. The third therapist referred to the possibility of creating near the client on a separate page or drawing objects or any other content related to the student's artwork, sometimes in consultation with the student. The images can be cut out, and then handed to the student who can decide whether to use them and where to paste them. Finally, one of the interviewees emphasized how important it is not to push "togetherness". In her view, the art therapist should primarily be present and responsive enough to eventually be incorporated into the artwork.

The open studio

One art therapist described an open studio she runs in conjunction with an occupational therapist in a special school for students with moderate-to-low-functioning ASD. They debated how to organize the studio to elicit creativity but not overwhelm the students with too many stimuli. They recruited six students, one from each class, mostly those who connected to art or whom the staff thought they might benefit from an encounter with art materials. They arranged the art materials on a marble surface with the standard materials in one corner (gouache, modeling clay, pencils, paints, etc.) and variable materials in another corner (materials from nature, all kinds of found objects, etc.). Each week they collected the students from their classrooms. This itself encouraged students to learn to knock on the door and ask a group member to come with them. The beginning and end of the session were spent together around the table. In most of the sessions, however, the work was free, and students could work around the shared table or in separate areas for personal creative work. The art therapist described the communication that emerged between the students. Through shape and color, they expressed their mode of observing and processing the works of the group members. The students literally studied each other and expressed it in the artwork. At the end of each session, the group facilitators took the time to process and write down their impressions of the experience, which further sharpened the in-depth observation of the processes the students engaged in.

Group art therapy

Group art therapy for students with ASD not only has considerable potential to improve social skills that can be generalized to other environments, but also enables them to form friendships by acquiring social skills in groups (Epp, 2008). Epp (2008) conducted groups for six participants with ASD. The encounter was divided into several parts. First, the group met for refreshments. The group then had a ten-minute structured group discussion that included guiding questions about events related to each student's day before the group session. This was followed by 30 minutes of guided creation that typically required interaction between group members, and finally, 20 minutes of free time for creation and play. D'Amico and Lalonde (2017) also described a group of six clients. The art therapists devised a variety of activities for the students to cooperate and to build group cohesion. In one, they encouraged them to build a tower using newspaper, tape, and string, which was followed by a discussion about their experience of working together, including the challenges as well as the positive and pleasurable aspects of working as a group.

One of the interviewees described the construction of a joint space during group artwork. Within this space, each student always has a personal space as well. The work alternates between the personal space and the joint space, while trying to expand the students' ability to engage in play. Another therapist noted that at times in groups of students with ASD, the children spread out in the room but still express something of themselves. From a group perspective, she felt it was important to pay attention to each student's voice as well as the group voice. The way in which concepts from the group world are presented in the session is specific to this population and sometimes requires efforts at comprehension on the part of the therapist. Another model described by one of the art therapists involved treating a pair of middle- or low-functioning students along with the two art therapists who had worked with them for several years. Meeting with the familiar faces of the therapists helped expand the students' circle of communication.

A group-class art therapy model

Since special education classes for students with ASD are usually small, the class teacher and assistant can at times join in a group-class activity (see Chapter 1). One art therapist noted that this format is useful especially in cases where the staff takes a very rigid didactic position toward a student with behavioral problems, whereas the art therapist tries to better understand the dynamic meaning of the student's behavior. In this model, the staff is invited to work together so that each behavior can be observed and understood in depth. The therapeutic-emotional work consists of using the art materials in a classroom setting. The art therapist can select a topic for this type of group. For example, one of the art therapists talked about therapeutic work based on songs that the students loved, that also included art. In lower functioning groups, for example, the art therapist can encourage work on feelings and senses, to which the students can connect emotions (for example a tactile box that contains an art material where students feel the material and discover it slowly and then can create with it). She said that in her group class, she organizes the activities and reflects the emotional parts, while the class teacher and assistant support the students in the more behavioral aspects. At the end of each session, time is devoted to a staff conversation and a summary of the session.

Another art therapist who also works with middle- and lower-functioning students described a slightly different structure. At the beginning of the session, the group listens to their regular class song (which is often related to the class goal). The song is usually accompanied by movements. Then, several art material stations are opened up. The stations cater to the interests and preferences of the students and they can choose and play with them. One of her goals is to expose the staff to the emotional sides of each student. In the first sessions, the team mostly observes and does not intervene. During the sessions, the art therapist teaches the staff how to reflect different behaviors to the students. This process helps staff members better understand these students' emotional experiences. For example, an educator who came in when a student was under the table went under the table herself and suddenly realized his need to be there. In staff meetings at the beginning of the process, everyone simply describes what they observed about each student. After a few sessions, they assign these observations so that each staff member observes two students. During the observation, they reflect their behaviors to the students and later their perceptions of their emotions. The therapist said that the students are eager to hear their names called and listen to the description of what they were doing.

Parent–child art psychotherapy

In kindergartens and the lower classes, parent–child art psychotherapy is sometimes recommended. In these situations, the parents come to the educational framework and take part in the treatment session together with their child. These therapies focus primarily on working on the relationship and communication between parent and child.

Self-advocacy

One art therapist described her work on self-advocacy primarily with students with higher-functioning ASD. Because ASD is an invisible difference, these students are often misunderstood or rejected by their classmates (in integrated classrooms) who do not grasp what causes them to have different behaviors. These students often feel estranged from their classmates. At times, this stems from the fact that they leave class to go to therapy or a reinforcement class and sometimes they themselves realize that they struggle to understand social situations, humor, different interests, etc. Students studying in a special education class integrated into a regular school are sometimes sensitive to the specificity of their class that has fewer students, more staff, and class hours through to the afternoon and on holidays. Self-advocacy helps these students understand their own differences and become more aware and self-accepting as well as upfront with this difference. As a result, in most cases, students with ASD acquire a better understanding and are accepted better by their classmates and peers.

Working with students on self-advocacy must be coordinated with working with their parents, who should be full partners and initiate discussions with their children about their differences, the diagnosis, and connect them to other individuals with ASD. This process is not always straightforward because some parents find it difficult to talk to their child about the diagnosis, whether out of the parents' inability to accept the diagnosis, but often out of fear that talking about the diagnosis will lead to rejection of the child by the environment. The process begins with the definition and conceptualization of the student's abilities and difficulties in various environments (home, educational, and therapeutic). Next, the art therapist, together with the student, defines areas of interest/abilities and difficulties/areas of knowledge specific to the student while paying special attention to communication skills specific to the student such as good memory, a well-developed imagination, visual ability, rigidity and repetition, difficulty in transitions, etc. This process can be depicted visually on a graph or cards, or through artwork. Next, the parents initiate a discussion with the child, in which they give the child's characteristics a diagnostic label and talk to the child about the diagnosis. After the conceptualization by the parents and then within the therapeutic process, work also begins on developing ever-widening circles which involve emotional processing with both the student and parents, acquaintances with individuals who have ASD (model figures), and then sharing the diagnosis with a respected educational figure and finally with the rest of the class. This process can be done within individual therapy, but also within a group context. In a group context, it is also possible to observe the commonalities between students.

THE MEANING OF ART

The study (Regev & Snir, 2013) on the contribution of art materials to working with students with ASD yielded a number of key points which were developed by the ten expert art therapists who took part. These are detailed below.

Art – An additional channel of communication

Most participants indicated that clients typically had difficulty communicating, which occasionally was accompanied by a language deficiency. As a result, the content areas available for discussion were restricted, as was the ability to handle emotions. In this context, the interviewees viewed the creative dimension as a realm that enabled communication and self-expression.

Art materials – A means of sensory activation

Most art therapists emphasized the importance of working initially with regressive art materials, as well as with para-art materials such as water, sand, and dough in sessions with ASD children in the pre-symbolic stage. The basic sensations of pouring and palpating can elicit the child's curiosity and activate the child's senses. The materials enable the child to experience cause and effect and to encounter the world through the senses.

Pleasure from artistic activity leads to session engagement

Therapy sessions, as described by the majority of the art therapists, were intrinsically repetitive, and occasionally characterized by a complete absence of activity; in this context, the positive experience of the sensory encounter with the art materials helped engage the child with ASD in creative activity. As a result, the child remained focused on the session and within the limits of the assigned space, through elicitation of curiosity and a sense of pleasure.

Art as a third-party mediator in the client-therapist relationship

The artistic activity in which the client and therapist are immersed becomes a third party in the art therapy room that mediates between them by reducing the threat of direct, face-to-face intimacy. The art materials, as objects (opposed to living things), are perceived by the children as non-threatening, and they are less anxious about engaging with them.

Art draws clients out of the autistic bubble

The sensory qualities of the art materials, the colors, scents, sounds, and tangible textures make them appealing and inviting, thus eliciting the clients' curiosity. In this sense, the materials can not only encourage interaction but also create the motivation to open a window onto the world and reach out from the autistic bubble.

Art provides a controllable environment (where the client can simply be)

Preserved art materials, such as pencils, markers, or chalk, were described by some of the art therapists as a particularly good match for some students with ASD, because these materials have a passive and static quality, thus providing the clients with a safe and controllable environment. In this way, the students can cope with their anxiety without feeling threatened within this environment.

The artistic product helps create continuity

Students with ASD often have difficulties with symbolism, which in turn has a deleterious effect on their ability to perceive any type of continuity; e.g., the continuity of events, memories, or associations. Since artistic activity leaves an actual trace in the form of a product that can be preserved and returned to at a later time, it helps create a sense of continuity. The artistic product becomes the palpable connection between one session and the next, in a process that helps develop the capacity for symbolism.

Art records and helps create a notion of self-presence

In some of the interviews, the art therapists mentioned that within the creative process, as students leave a mark of their own artwork on the page, the wall, or in the room, the artistic product becomes a record of their presence within the space.

Art helps increase the clients' range of patterns

The majority of the interviewees noted that one of the main functions of the use of art is to prompt additional patterns. This broadening of the repertoire can take the form of the way the material was used or the children's ability to vary, enrich, and develop a narrative through a repeated image.

A number of interviewees addressed the importance of art therapy as provided in the education system for these students. Since in class they are required to behave in a certain way that includes studying and proper conduct, they actually have to work very, very hard all the time. In art therapy, they can relax. The art therapy room is a containing place that accepts them as they are. It is a place where they do not need to "achieve". Touching the material becomes an authentic experience and an opportunity for self-expression and empowerment.

COLLABORATIVE INTERVENTIONS INVOLVING PARENTS AND STAFF MEMBERS

The literature suggests that consistency on the part of parents, teachers, and therapists is one of the key ways to help students with ASD (Emery, 2004).

Working with parents

Encounters with parents in the educational system in Israel usually take place three times a year and are mainly intended to update the parents on their children's status, behavior, and progress and for the art therapists to be updated on the situation at home. One interviewee felt that there is not always enough contact with parents and that much closer cooperation is needed. As the student gets older, the nature of this dialogue shifts. Whereas at the beginning, the diagnosis and the impact of being the parent of a child with ASD tend to be addressed to a greater extent, later parents may want to deal with the issue of involving the child in the diagnosis and in what way. One art therapist described how she helps parents tell their children, usually relatively high-functioning students, that they have characteristics typical of people with ASD. Sometimes this process takes years until the parents agree to indeed talk to their child about the diagnosis. In addition, parents may need help to deal with bureaucratic issues such as HMOs, finding the appropriate educational framework, and the move to a hostel after graduation, etc. On the other hand, a number of art therapists, mostly those working with middle- and lower-functioning students, discussed efforts to engage with parents. They noted that they find it difficult to recruit parents who are exhausted after years of coping to come to school for therapeutic work and parental guidance.

One art therapist emphasized the importance throughout the treatment of gathering information from the parents. She uses this information as part of her sessions with the student. For example, she asks parents what they did over the weekend or what happened on a particular holiday. The art therapist thus looks for ways to help students talk about themselves using the information she has learned from the parents.

More than with other populations in special education, almost all the art therapists emphasized the importance of multidisciplinary team-work. The staff members define the goals together and all of them work together, as a function of the field, to advance these goals. For instance, although the group-class model was run differently by different art therapists, all concurred that its purpose was to expose the educational staff to the students' emotional world. Some art therapists stressed the importance of developing the educational staff's capabilities to engage in a deeper, dynamic understanding of the students' emotional world.

CLINICAL ILLUSTRATION

Tali, age 13, was born with moderate-functioning ASD, barely speaks, and is sometimes assisted by alternative supportive communication. She is the only daughter of relatively older parents. She attends a special school for students with moderate and low-functioning ASD. There are seven students in her class. Because she loves colors and paintings, Tali was included in an innovative open studio project at her school. Her educator told her that on a given Sunday the art therapist would come to pick her up for a session with other students where she could draw. It was difficult for the educator to understand from her reaction whether she was pleased to join the group.

On Sunday, there was a knock on the classroom door and the art therapist stood in the doorway. She went up to Tali and invited her to come with her to the art therapy room. Tali went with her and, on the way, they picked up a number of other students from other classes. When they got to the art therapy room, the art materials had already been set out on a long table by the wall. Tali went over and arranged them the way she likes them to be, according to the colors of the rainbow. The art therapist asked her to sit down, explained to all the students the rules of the room and suggested they take paints and start creating. Tali stayed seated. She didn't seem quite sure what to do.

The art therapist then asked her to come with her. Tali got up hesitantly. They went to the buffet together and looked at the art materials.

There were all kinds of materials and it seemed that Tali was having a hard time choosing what to work with. The art therapist suggested a basket of oil chalks. Together they went to a joint table on which sheets of paper had been laid out. Tali sat down with the sheet and colors in front of her. Tali stayed seated while the art therapist continued to move among the students. A few minutes passed. Tali sat quietly. She took out the colors and arranged them in her favorite order again. Then she sat quietly again. Out of the corner of her eye, she saw Avner drawing a large yellow sun. This sun caught her attention and she watched with interest how Avner smeared the colors and how the yellows and reds and oranges blended into each other. With a hesitant hand, Tali also took yellow paint and began to draw delicate circles in the corner of her page.

A week later, the next Sunday, the art therapist came again to pick up Tali from the classroom to go to the art therapy room. This time Tali went over herself and took a pack of markers and went to the joint table. This time, too, Tali looked around. Dana was right in front of her. She was working in watercolors and was letting green-blue paint stains spread on her drawing that mingled with each other. Every touch by Dana on the page produced a new world of stains. Tali was fascinated. She rearranged her colors and also chose shades of green-blue. She tried to combine them in her own way. While drawing with great concentration, suddenly she saw another work by Yaniv made up of sharp black lines that intersected each other. This image also fascinated her. Her eyes wandered between Dana's merging colors and Yaniv's sharp shafts. Dana's colors looked like swirling seawater. Yaniv's prongs looked like thorns or swords. She incorporated both images and her page began to fill with green-blue spots, but also sharp black lines that cut across the page.

Tali continued to come to the art therapy room every week. When the art therapist knocked on the door, she would immediately get up and go with her, and it was obvious how eager she was for these sessions. She hardly spoke in the open studio, but she watched the colors and shapes produced by the other students in the group care-fully. Each session she summarized the sights she saw, that always incorporated lines, spots, shapes, and images of the works in her spe-cial way that showed that she acknowledged the students working around her and allowed their works to be processed through her.

SUMMARY

This chapter presented a number of goals. The prime goal of working in art therapy with students with ASD is to develop contact and communication, where art materials can provide an additional language for expression. Art therapy also helps in behavioral, sensory, and emotional regulation. The feel of the art materials can help induce calm, and the wide range of possibilities of working with art materials in different ways and textures can help expand the students' range of possibilities without flooding them with anxiety. Through art, students can also begin to represent their experiences and tell their personal stories. This serves to expand the symbolic space and opens up new possibilities for communication. This communication can also defuse stressful and anxious situations, such as transitions between educational frameworks. Finally, for higher-functioning students, art therapy can enable them to observe their evolving identity as individuals with ASD.

Alongside these objectives, a number of challenges were mentioned. The first challenge is the extreme heterogeneity in the students' mode of communication. Art therapists who have worked with this population for years note that previous experience does not prepare them for the next client because apart from general traits, the communication patterns, interests, and emotional difficulties of each student need to be explored in depth. They also need to deal with the specific dilemma of therapy in the education system; namely, whether to encourage students to venture out of the autistic bubble, because the art therapy room can actually serve as a place where these students can let down their guard rather than be under pressure to constantly interact with others. Some of the art therapists noted the difficulties relating to clients' rigidity and repetitiveness. This difficulty may also affect the building of the therapeutic alliance. They also noted that behavioral problems, even when not expressed within the art therapy room, often penetrate the therapeutic bubble through the systemic work itself, which may complicate the therapeutic encounter. Finally, they used terms such as "emptiness", "unnecessary", and "non-existent" to describe their sense of being ignored at certain moments in the treatment, which constantly challenges the therapeutic relationship.

The interventions proposed in this chapter can be divided into three main groups. The first covers interventions designed to help the student cope with difficulties. This involves finding ways to deal with sensory regulation through the specific ways of introducing art materials (e.g., clay in a plastic bag), proposing calming techniques (e.g., mandalas) and sensory work where the art product is secondary to the experience. To deal with repetition and rigidity, the art materials can provide expansions as can combining elements of play, movement, and music with the artwork. The second group covers interventions designed to help the student tell his or her story. The work can promote the development of the symbolic world and allow for the representation of personal experiences. Through comics, social stories, or a visual diary, these experiences begin to take shape. They can also help the students look at themselves as a person with ASD and promote self-advocacy. The third group covers interventions designed to increase the students' connection and communication with their immediate environment. This can be done through working on joint drawings together or on separate sheets of paper, in an open studio where students are invited to create freely side by side, and through group work including the group-class model and parent–child art psychotherapy.

REFERENCES

Alter-Muri, S. B. (2017). Art education and art therapy strategies for autism spectrum disorder students. *Art Education, 70*(5), 20–25.

Alvarez, A., Reid, S., et al. (1999). *Autism and personality: Findings from the Tavistock Autism Workshop.* Routledge.

Bion, W. R. (1994). *Learning from experience.* Jason Aronson.

D'Amico, M., & Lalonde, C. (2017). The effectiveness of art therapy for teaching social skills to children with autism spectrum disorder. *Art Therapy, 34*(4), 176–182.

Emery, M. J. (2004). Art therapy as an intervention for autism. *Art Therapy, 21*(3), 143–147.

Epp, K. M. (2008). Outcome-based evaluation of a social skills program using art therapy and group therapy for children on the autism spectrum. *Children & Schools, 30*(1), 27–36.

Evans, K., & Dubowski, J. (2001). *Art therapy with children on the autistic spectrum: Beyond words.* Jessica Kingsley.

Gazeas, M. (2012). Current findings on art therapy and individuals with autism spectrum disorder. *Canadian Art Therapy Association Journal, 25*(1), 15–22.

Grandin, T. (2008). *Thinking in pictures, expanded edition: My life with autism.* Vintage.

Martin, N. (2008). Assessing portrait drawings created by children and adolescents with autism spectrum disorder. *Journal of the American Art Therapy Association, 25*(1), 15–23.

Martin, N. (2009). Art therapy and autism: Overview and recommendations. *Art Therapy*, 26(4), 187–190.

Osborne, J. (2003). Art and the Child with Autism: Therapy or education? *Early Child Development and Care*, 173(4), 411–423.

Regev, D., & Snir, S. (2013). Art therapy for treating children with Autism Spectrum Disorders (ASD): The unique contribution of art materials. *The Academic Journal of Creative Arts Therapies*, 3(2), 251–260.

Schweizer, C., Knorth, E. J., & Spreen, M. (2014). Art therapy with children with Autism Spectrum Disorders: A review of clinical case descriptions on 'what works'. *The Arts in Psychotherapy*, 41(5), 577–593.

Schweizer, C., Knorth, E. J., van Yperen, T. A., & Spreen, M. (2019). Consensus-based typical elements of art therapy with children with autism spectrum disorders. *International Journal of Art Therapy*, 24(4), 181–191.

Scheuermann, B., & Webber, J. (2002). *Autism: Teaching does make a difference*. Wadsworth.

Van Lith, T., Stallings, J. W., & Harris, C. E. (2017). Discovering good practice for art therapy with children who have Autism Spectrum Disorder: The results of a small scale survey. *The Arts in Psychotherapy*, 54, 78–84.

BRIEF BIOGRAPHIES OF THE ART THERAPISTS WHO CONTRIBUTED TO THIS CHAPTER

Einat Bibi, art therapist (M.A.) and supervisor, has worked for 22 years as an art therapist with kindergarten children and students with ASD.

Sivan Eyal, art therapist (M.A.) and supervisor, has worked for 13 years in the education system, including 6 years as an art therapist with students with ASD.

Yael Guterman, art therapist (M.A.) and supervisor, has worked for 30 years with children with ASD including 22 years as an art therapist and supervisor specialist in ASD in the education system.

Nily Kairy, art therapist (M.A.) and supervisor, has worked for 28 years in the education system, including 20 years as an art therapist with students with ASD.

Revital Rada, art therapist (M.A.), has worked for six years as an art therapist in the education system with students with ASD.

Tamar Sade-Dor, art therapist (M.A.) and supervisor, has worked for 22 years in the education system, including 13 years as an art therapist with students with ASD.

Revital Turiski, art therapist (M.A.) and supervisor, has worked for 12 years as an art therapist in the education system, including 4 years with students with ASD.

Five

INTRODUCTION

Intellectual and developmental disabilities (IDD) are characterized by considerable deficits in cognitive, functional, and adaptive life skills, with an IQ score of 70 or below. People with IDD generally tend to have difficulty expressing their thoughts and feelings verbally, which increases the likelihood that they will display their emotions through maladaptive behaviors that can disrupt social relationships (Ho et al., 2020).

Students with IDD are often oriented toward art therapy for a variety of emotional disorders that sometimes result from a dual morbidity. These students tend to be exposed to far more vulnerabilities and traumas than the general population, which often complicates their interactions with others and their surroundings. One of the art therapists interviewed here emphasized that today almost all the clients with IDD she treats have experienced some kind of trauma in their lives. Throughout this chapter, the art therapists emphasize the impact of different levels of functioning, which affects ways of working with this population. In the case of very low functioning clients, art therapy in fact incorporates hardly any art.

White et al. (2009) noted that early approaches to working with clients with IDD in art therapy involved centering primarily around the notion of "art as therapy". More recent approaches consider that it is also possible to work more dynamically with these clients. According to Lett (2005), two approaches are considered to be the most beneficial in the treatment of individuals with IDD. The first is developmental art therapy, which treats an individual in reference to his or her developmental progression. This approach to art is based on the notion of cognitive, emotional, and artistic maturation. Typical development is used as a yardstick for treatment. The second is behavioral

DOI: 10.4324/9781003156918-5

art therapy, which is designed to treat observed undesirable behavior through the application of behavior modification techniques as part of the art therapy process.

Ashby (2011) surveyed 60 art therapists working with people with severe IDD displaying challenging behavior in the UK. The therapists reported that they believed they had provided a wide range of benefits to people with severe IDD and challenging behavior. More specifically, they considered their approaches effective if they provided safety and containment, empowerment, a thinking space to reflect and process, and an opportunity to develop a meaningful and trusting relationship. The art therapists also felt that they played a role in enhancing communication through the development of non-verbal skills by modifying and re-directing challenging behavior into more positive outlets of expression. Nevertheless, defining the therapeutic goals of art therapy for this population can vary considerably.

THE THERAPEUTIC GOALS OF ART THERAPY

The advantage of art therapy in general, as compared to other treatments, is that the artistic process allows individuals to experience a therapeutic setting without the typical verbal expectations (Trzaska, 2012). Art therapists often note that one of the goals of therapy is to enable the expression of a wide range of emotions through artwork which may be hard to convey in words. This includes negative emotions, which can be given a place and expression in the art therapy room.

The interviewees here repeatedly raised the issue of the defensive repetition and obsessive behaviors these clients often implement to reduce anxiety. In art therapy, this emerges for example when a student executes the same work week after week. The goal of art therapy in this case is to expand the realm of possibilities. One art therapist commented that individuals with IDD tend to manifest a very limited range of possibilities. The goal is thus to expand this range and allow for more emotions and behaviors to come to the fore, which are expressed, through a gradual and mediated process that increases the range of creative materials and techniques clients use to create and present in their works. In this way, confidence in the art therapy room is maintained, the obsession is moderated, and repetition is reduced and sometimes disappears.

Another issue has to do with regulation. One art therapist noted that there is often no middle ground in these students in terms of emotional and behavioral regulation: there is either much too much or much too little behavior, so that the goal of art therapy is to achieve a greater balance.

Art was described by a number of the art therapists as access to a new world for these students. They saw their role as developing creativity and allowing for it to be expressed in the art therapy room in a way that affects these students' feelings of competence. This can foster change in other facets of their lives. One art therapist argued that since the clients' images are often related to the concrete world, part of art therapy also involves an attempt to develop the world of the imagination, the symbolic world, at least for students who are capable of this. This includes being able to play or fantasize and start grasping the difference between play and reality.

Another art therapist underscored the goal of creating a meaningful relationship. Students with IDD who have experienced years of being traumatized and rejected in complex relationships first need to learn to trust and feel accepted as complete human beings. A close, intimate relationship is formed with the art therapist that allows students to behave authentically and express themselves in different ways, knowing that they will not be judged. In higher functioning clients, art therapy can promote the capacity for mentalization, leading to the realization that the behavior of those around them stems from and is influenced by others' inner worlds. Through dialogue with the art therapist, students learn to understand their own inner worlds. After years of therapy and observation, this can lead to a better grasp of others and their ideas, and the similarities and differences from their own.

The art therapists also addressed the important goal of creating a place where the student meets an adult in a one-on-one relationship that includes acceptance and inclusion. In the art therapy room, students are encouraged to evolve in an accepting and non-judgmental atmosphere. This aspect according to the interviewees is extremely significant for the students. One interviewee stressed how important it is not to set any goals but simply allow these clients to be in an enabling space, where experiences that are difficult for them to articulate elsewhere can resonate, including experiences of emotional injury.

One art therapist working with higher functioning students argued that one of the main goals of art therapy is to help them be aware of their strengths and weaknesses and develop a kind of reality that fulfills their strengths, but also takes their difficulties and limitations into account. In art therapy, clients can sometimes enter into fantasy worlds, but they eventually need to return to reality and not sink into depression and despair where they feel incompetent. In addition, art therapy strengthens their ability to enter a transitional space in therapy between fantasy and reality and make entering and exiting it outside of therapy easier. When students reach the age of 21 and have to leave school, this recognition of what they are capable of and what they are unable to do on their own as an adult is often cultivated within therapy, especially in higher functioning students.

Another art therapist noted that within the treatment the students begin to learn who they are as people: What do they like? What do they dislike? What do they want for themselves? This is related to issues of self-construction and independence, which should also be addressed with their parents. It is also linked to the ability to know how to ask for and receive help when needed and to present their strengths and weaknesses to others. Sometimes independence can generate emotional obstacles such as anxiety, or the fear of being manipulated or making decisions alone. These steps toward independence can be explored and rehearsed in art therapy through mentalization processes. Another goal especially for higher functioning students is learning to make choices. This can start with the choice of the creative materials in the art therapy room and lead to more significant choices in the student's life, depending on their abilities and level of functioning.

Finally, one of the art therapists working with low-functioning students emphasized how important it is for art therapists to be able to express the students' voice even outside the art therapy room. In the art therapy room, new attitudes, feelings, and capabilities or frustrations are sometimes revealed, and it is important for this information to be mediated to the staff. For example, sometimes a student's smile does not necessarily express joy, or banging on the desk does not necessarily express anger or frustration. In this respect, art therapy in special education and especially with low-functioning students is very different from classical art therapy in which everything that happens in the therapy room is kept confidential.

CHALLENGES

Art therapy for students with IDD is slow and the changes are small and unfold in miniscule increments. Comments such as "frustration", "boredom", and "fatigue" came up in many interviews as counter-transference challenges. Art therapists often experience a sense of isolation in the art therapy room when students are low functioning or have dual diagnoses involving Autism Spectrum Disorder (ASD) that makes contact very difficult. This is also true outside the therapy room since there are so few art therapists who specialize in this population. In addition, the interviewees cited these clients' lack of initiative and the difficulty of being with students who constantly have to be motivated to do something. The art therapists mentioned needing the patience to stick with situations where no change is taking place, and still be able to believe in movement and change. A number of interviewees noted that this slow process required a great deal of internal work from them which involved honing their ability to see small changes and learning to be satisfied and see the benefits in them.

During the interviews, a number of art therapists discussed their negative reactions when they first encountered IDD students. One issue was hygiene, including students who drool because they have low muscle tone. One art therapist said she initially actually went through a transition ritual when she came home to rid herself of the experiences in the art therapy room, so that they did not spill over to her private life and family. However, this same therapist said that with time, her empathy increased, and she now cherishes these students once she gets to know them better.

Another interviewee noted that young low functioning IDD students can sometimes discover what deters and frightens the staff and use this behavior to manipulate them and get their attention. For example, one student took off his diaper and smeared its contents. Another student stripped naked, after realizing that it shocked the people around her. For the art therapist, these are extremely challenging moments, but also contain the seeds of change because precisely within the contained art therapy room, it is possible to be a little less frightened and convey a different message in response to these behaviors. In addition, in these situations, an additional staff member can be called in for assistance. One of the interviewees said that she asks the staff members for help in these difficult situations and holds several meetings with them after the incident to give them an opportunity to express and process the event.

One of the art therapists also described the frustration that emerges when the staff considers that the student could be given more independence, but the parents are opposed. In this case, the art therapist and the staff feel they have missed an opportunity after having invested in the student. This therapist noted that she talks to parents about possibilities for independent life when their children are still very young to give them time to get used to the idea of independence. Disagreements with parents can also revolve around a comprehensive diagnosis or medication, where the therapist and the staff may feel that the parents are hindering the student's potential.

INTERVENTION TECHNIQUES AND DEDICATED WORKING MODELS

This section details interventions and models from the literature and considerations gleaned from the interviews. The differences in opinions and intervention techniques among art therapists here were much greater for IDD students than for the other disabilities described in the previous chapters. These mainly emerged in terms of the scope of intervention of the art therapist and the extent to which direct guidance of the student is used (perhaps reflective of the differences between the developmental approach and the behavioral approach presented in the introduction). The art therapists who chose to intervene less argued that what was important was inclusion and admiration, the ability to see the clients in a new perspective because they, unlike their parents, have chosen to work with this population. In their view, this approach can lead to change and progress. The art therapists who believed in greater intervention suggested a variety of ways to do so. One art therapist noted that the level of intervention is also related to the level of functioning and that she may shift between less or more intervention depending on the specific student.

Flexibility on the part of the art therapist

The issue of flexibility in art therapy came up in almost all the interviews. Flexibility covers a very wide range of behaviors. Sometimes it involves leaving the art therapy room and going outside with the student because this is the most appropriate for this specific client at a specific time. According to one of the interviewees, a great deal can be done with students individually: what guides her is their current condition and what they need from her. Accordingly, she will sometimes take walks with students, cook with them, and sometimes do artwork with them. The art process can also sometimes include creating for the client, and acting as his/her extension, but out of a real understanding that this is what s/he needs at that moment. Another interviewee said that she considers flexibility to be the most important parameter and sometimes goes outside the art therapy room especially after transitions, for example with seventh graders who are entering middle school and need time to adapt to the new setting. One of the art therapists who works in kindergartens said that for these children, the initial intervention will often take place in the kindergarten classroom before gradually moving to the art therapy room. In kindergarten, she takes one child at a time, but the effect percolates to the other children as well. The initial relationship is like a mother–baby interaction with many peek-a-boo games. Later she offers choices in certain situations and reflects to the child what is allowed and what is not.

Flexibility also requires the art therapist to prepare for a broad spectrum of art making from pre-creation such as mixing all kinds of art materials and creating various potions to concrete and symbolic artwork. One of the interviewees said that sometimes even very basic mother–child contact activities take place such as concretely giving the student a hot drink and a cookie or helping disheveled students with their personal hygiene by combing their hair or washing their hands. Another art therapist described her efforts to find an optimal form of treatment for these clients by addressing their needs and their primal traumas. A number of therapists noted that they sometimes incorporate other arts including movement, musical instruments, songs, and other modalities into art therapy. According to them, especially with students who behave in an obsessive way, movement, for example, can be very liberating and can open the door to art making.

Interventions using art materials

Some art therapists emphasized how they intervene in art making by suggesting a particular material, technique, or instrument. For example, one student had trouble regulating the amount of paint she was using so that at the end of the session the room looked like a battlefield. The intervention with her was to help her regulate how much paint she would prepare. This was done as a game, where one of them poured the paint into a recipient and the other would say when it was enough. This developmental transition from work in very primary and basic materials, especially in students with very significant basic deficits, to more mature work, can take years.

The interventions often start with a topic that interests the student (e.g., a singer the student admires) and from there expands to other issues more closely related to self-expression. One of the art therapists described an intervention where she asked a student to draw himself on a very large sheet of paper, as a form of empowerment and as a way to engage in a more long-term complex project. The therapist also stressed the need for in-depth knowledge of the art materials and their potential uses. For example, gouache can be used in a variety of ways, from regressive to fairly reserved, and the intervention should be tailored to each client. The same developmental transition from primary regressive material to more controlled material can also constitute a mode of working in the same session based on clinical/dynamic theory which suggests that after satisfying initial needs and releasing impulses, the client can engage in more controlled materials and create a more structured and developed piece of work. Working in this format can help the client emerge from the session feeling more structured and with a heightened sense of ability.

One of the interviewees described how he introduces students to the art materials and their possibilities. In each session, he suggests different materials and different emotional expressions. All refer to abstract artwork that expresses emotions such as anger or fear. Thus, students learn in the first months of art therapy that they can work in a wide range of materials and harness them for emotional expression. If they are really interested in this type of work, they learn to enjoy it, play with it, and express themselves through it. Later, students can be allowed to choose what they want to do because they are already familiar with the materials and options for expression and are not afraid of them.

A number of art therapists emphasized the importance of working with gouache paints with IDD students, although their techniques varied. One described the advantages of using a gouache table with a goblet and a brush for each color. The student learns how to take a different color each time and go from the gouache table to the paper pinned to the wall. According to her, working in this way encourages the creation of a series of paintings and a great deal of deepening and development in creative work, which also has a positive effect on everyday life. By contrast, another art therapist teaches IDD students to use only one brush that needs to be rinsed between colors. Her experience indicates that even lower functioning students can learn this technique and can enjoy exploring and developing flexibility when they discover that color mixes with color or color mixes with water.

Work with repetition

All the art therapists without exception described repetitive situations where the students repeat the same artwork or the same narrative over and over again. The interviewees, all of whom have extensive experience in the field, nevertheless took different approaches to repetition. One interviewee stated that she reflects this back to the student verbally, but at times also concretely by placing a specific object on the table each time there is a repetition. Over time, the students become aware of the repetition which can be related to when it arises.

Some described how they decide to intervene either by saying that they are now doing something else, or by changing the substrate or material. One art therapist said she recently started using a sensory water table in situations where she felt there was no movement in therapy, and that water play helped make the session more lively. Another interviewee described a group session where there was repetition from the participants. In response, he asked all the participants to take out five to seven artworks and choose the one that they liked best and put the rest back in the folder. Then, each of them was asked to hand the artwork to the person on their right. The students were then asked to copy their seatmate's work as best they could. This process gave the participants a glimpse into another participant's life, empathy, as well as exposure to a new experience. Based on the success of this approach, he started to show individual students, artists' abstract artworks which they then attempted to copy.

Other art therapists were less inclined to intervene and argued that there was no point in fighting repetition since the full acceptance of the clients ultimately led to change. One art therapist indicated that she provides space for small changes to take place, which gradually enables students to move away from repetition on their own. Each time one of her students makes a change, she says: "Something new happened here" until gradually the students come to the studio asking to do something new.

Process of mirroring

One of the interviewees discussed the fact that after many years of working with these students, she realized that instead of signaling them out and telling them what they can and cannot do, she decided to let go and let them express themselves freely. She then imitates them and does what they do, which enables these students to perceive what they are experiencing. The imitation ("mirroring") helps convey that she is not frightened of the students and accepts them and their behavior, which gives the students a clear sense of "I am being observed" but also "I exist". This total acceptance by the art therapist can promote a sense of security. Imitation exists in many forms as well as in art. For example, instead of criticizing a student who painted off the sheet of paper, a tactic that halted the creative process, she imitated and also painted outside the boundaries of the page. She considers that mirroring strengthens the bond between therapist and student who often wait for her impatiently in class and ask about her during the week. Once she understands the student's artwork in depth, she can direct it toward a finished product. For example, one very low-functioning student barely managed to use her hands but did manage to squeeze paint out of a bottle. The color coming out, the squishing sound of the bottle, and the color on the paper gave her a lot of pleasure. The art therapist helped turn the paint into an artwork by folding the paper into a butterfly. At times the art therapist adds something beyond exact imitation, which kindles the students' curiosity.

Tal Goffer has developed a method of working with a transparent wheeled board she uses to give students the experience of leading and being led, working on portraits by facing each other, free work on both sides of the board, and sensory work. Students can work with gouache, markers, or colored foam. They work opposite each other, so they can see each other through the transparent board. The artwork involves highlighting the difference between transparent and opaque. This work, which deals with echoing, imitation, and observation, is suitable for both toddlers and older groups and gives students a sense of visibility. At the end of the activity, the students clean the board together.

Working with diaries

One art therapist described how she structures the therapeutic work with the students. Each client has a binder, and a new page is added to the binder each session. Each page is divided into four and each quarter has a reference to a specific aspect of the student's life that week: "an experience I had this week with friends/at school/at home..." or "a happy/sad/angry moment... that happened to me this week". One of the quarters can also be left free to draw or write. The diary, according to her, helps students tell their personal stories and express their feelings in a more structured way. The diaries constitute a framework, and the guidelines can range from clear and defined to fuzzy and open. Another art therapist works with visual diaries (see details in Chapter 4). In the diaries, the students can work with different art materials, different techniques, or integrate texts they like.

Integrating alternative supportive communication

Some art therapists described how they incorporate alternative forms of supportive communication into their work with students (using iPads or a visual focus system in which clients center their gaze on a word). This is done with language-delayed students to help them express themselves emotionally and to give them a broader range of choices. Some students benefit by being able to express content that otherwise could not be expressed. One of the therapists described how she articulates the emotion the student has chosen and helps him/her understand the meaning of a sentence by reframing: "When you point to a smile, it seems to me that you are happy and then I keep working with it; when you point to a nervous face, I understand we should change game now and do something else". She said that with all IDD students she starts and ends the session with a communication board and selects the appropriate emotions.

Using the cell phone in art therapy

One art therapist described how she used the students' cell phones to learn about their world. Students play songs they like for the therapist or show her YouTube videos. One student, for example, showed her videos about superheroes. This led to a talk about her powers and art making where the student made accessories for her role as a superheroine.

Open studio

Carrigan (1993) interviewed four Swiss art therapists who developed an open studio approach where clients only engage in painting. Each jar of color has its own brush. Participants can work with a brush or their fingers. The artwork is placed on an easel. There may not be any verbal processing by the art therapists, and the paintings are primarily a source of self-expression. When clients repeat the same artwork, they are allowed to do so until they reach saturation. The goal is for each client to spend time acquiring painting skills until they can express themselves through it. The artworks are kept in the studio and are the property of the artist. One of the interviewees, who runs an open studio at her school, emphasized the importance of displaying the products from the open studio in regular exhibits, to show what students can achieve to staff and families.

Another interviewee described the open studio in her school that is supervised by two co-therapists and sometimes is focused around one art material such as a papier-mâché workshop designed for students aged 15–21. Each student can choose what to make: a bowl, a statue, or work in relief. The work is free and aims to express the students' inner world. Another goal is to be able to work independently with the material, guided by the art therapist. Within the group, the participants choose where to work, the subject of the artwork, and their role in the group, such as being in charge of preparing the materials, helping others, or co-creating.

One of the interviewees also described an open studio that she runs together with an occupational therapist at a school. The goal is first and foremost to encourage independence in that each student chooses the art materials, the content of the work, and exactly where s/he will do it. The studio facilitators only try to show how to expand the creative process (the art therapist) and in what physical position the creative process will be the most comfortable and appropriate (the occupational therapist).

The issue of group work elicited numerous, very interesting comments. One art therapist described the wide variety of groups in the school composed of high-functioning IDD students. Some run throughout the school year and some are short-term. The groups are facilitated by a team made up of an arts therapist and another staff member and have five to an entire class of 12–15 students. The groups are either theme- or age-oriented. Some groups deal with a common theme, such as communication skills, social rejection, a group for adopted students, a family group (for students who have had difficult family experiences and can benefit from the experience of a family under the guidance of a female therapist and a male therapist). The age-related or school-related groups are for instance made up of seventh graders who just entered middle school. The goal of the group is to use creativity and play to help these students express their feelings about the transition and issues that arise in the classroom. Other groups for students aged 18–21 deal with issues such as interpersonal relationships. This type of dynamic group aims to strengthen their ability to talk about themselves, connect with others, and process issues before leaving the educational framework.

Another art therapist described groups of up to four students or whole classes that are run jointly with the educator in a school for lower functioning students. Since it is not easy for these students to stay active, she starts each group by having each student choose a sheet of paper and an oil chalk stick and make circles that can be small, large, bold, or faint while listening to music. This initial exercise helps them begin the session more calmly. During the sessions, if the students are able to do so, she works on group processes that continue over a number of sessions of transition from individual to group work. Within the group, they learn to wait, to restrain themselves (delay gratification), and to work together. However, in cases where she feels that the group is less relaxed and cannot work together, she switches to an open studio model, where each student works individually with the material they have chosen and presents the artwork to the others at the end of the session. The specific content and approach are tailored to each group.

Yet another art therapist stressed that after many years of working in teams, they found that individual art therapy with younger, lower-functioning students was far less effective than multidisciplinary group work. Therefore, they initiated a multidisciplinary work model in which staff members from different fields do group work together. For the most part, an art therapist, physiotherapist, educator, and assistant work with a small group of students so that almost all the students have an adult by their side. The student–adult dyads change from session to session. Within the session, there are transitions between different fields. This model has the advantage of enabling more holistic work, which contributes to students' progress. It also serves as modeling for the educator and the assistant who learn to introduce more therapeutic language into their educational work.

The fourth art therapist described a "safety" group for students aged 16 and over. The goal of the group was to learn to identify dangers and keep themselves safe both online and in the real world. Using art, cards, and narratives, the students described their experiences in a variety of places such as on public transportation or when walking to the mall. They also learned what to do when they identified a danger. For example, one activity in art was drawing their bodies, to identify feelings in different organs.

Some schools implement different models concurrently. In one school, some groups adhere to the principles of group-class art therapy. The assistants and the educator take part in these groups with the students. This model places the educator and assistants within the therapeutic circle, as participants. Together with the students, they are invited to express themselves through artwork and take part in the discussions. This is done to enable the staff to recharge their batteries and give the students another perspective on the group. Other groups in the same school revolve around a particular topic. For example, the art therapist conducted a group with a speech therapist and a visual impairment instructor. The focus was on students with IDD who also have visual impairments. The group setting made it possible for them to express the difficulties associated with their visual impairments for the first time. Each difficulty was eventually turned into a letter to the principal. This constituted a form of self-advocacy that was backed by the group facilitators. This letter resulted in improvements in accessibility for the visually impaired in the school (e.g., yellow communication signboards and special seating). Another group of female students worked on their femininity by discussing what is feminine, and where the students could experiment with activities that were less familiar to them such as nail polish or new hairstyles.

Verbal interventions

In the interviews, some art therapists emphasized the need to teach students who are able to communicate verbally how to observe and relate to their artwork. One art therapist noted that this process requires training the clients. He endeavors to make them part of the work (within the Gestalt approach) and present themselves as if they were specific characters or part of the artwork. He noted that one frequent theme is frustration from lack of contact. He attempts to provide an outlet for this frustration and also addresses the socio-sexual aspects of the student's identity. Another art therapist described her use of songs and trying to understand why a student chose a particular song and sharing her interpretation with the student.

THE MEANING OF ART

One art therapist described eureka moments when suddenly the student looks at his/her artwork, connects to it, and finds it beautiful. At these instants, the psyche blooms through the experience of success and ability which is so important for these students and becomes anchored within them.

Many art therapists described using art materials in a variety of ways to expand the students' range of expression, whether non-verbally or as a way to escape from repetition. Through interventions in art materials, new possibilities open up to them.

One interviewee emphasized that because students' ability to express themselves is enhanced through art materials and brings with it a new, richer expression that is unfamiliar to the student's environment, art therapists often organize exhibitions. These exhibitions constitute a source of pride, allow the staff and family members to rediscover aspects of their students/family members, and provide the students with an opportunity to communicate their strengths (as opposed to engaging with their disabilities) with others.

COLLABORATIVE INTERVENTIONS INVOLVING PARENTS AND STAFF MEMBERS

Working with parents

One of the art therapists emphasized how critical it is to work with the parents of these clients. Many parents of students with IDD find it hard to let their children be independent, which can lead to ongoing exchanges between the school staff and the parents. This is particularly true near graduation when parents need to allow their children to acquire as much independence as possible. The work with parents aims to convince them that independence is best for them and for their children.

Another interviewee noted that in her institution, parents dialogue with school staff in a variety of ways. Each art therapist is in direct contact with the students' parents. This involves meetings at least three times a year and phone calls as needed. Sometimes, at major milestones in the student's life, the parents are asked to meet with multidisciplinary staff members. In addition, certain parents receive parental guidance and may be asked to take part in parent–child art psychotherapy within the school setting. Finally, parents are encouraged to attend group workshops that generally last for 12 sessions and have 10–15 participants. The group works with therapeutic cards and through discussions. The content sometimes comes from the parents, but other topics are presented by the facilitators such as developmental stages, separation, and independence.

Working with staff members

Working within the school system or at an educational boarding school provides opportunities to observe students in all types of situations, including conflicts or misunderstandings with the staff. One art therapist mentioned that as part of her role she mediates conflict situations to allow the students to resume studying or calm down in the art therapy room. Since these frameworks are small and each student is under close observation, she can approach students outside of the therapy sessions to check whether they need help. Other therapists referred to working holistically with these students, and that they sometimes stay with them even outside of treatment such as during breaks or times when they feel the need and come to the art therapy room.

A number of art therapists addressed the creative forces inherent in these students. Facets of these students often emerge that are not seen outside the art therapy room. The art therapists hope to make others aware of these abilities by presenting artworks at the school to staff and parents so that they can acknowledge the students' achievements. Because many of these students have low ego functions, the role of the art therapist is to bring these achievements to the fore based on a dynamic grasp of the students' inner world. This can often lead to greater understanding on the part of the staff and can encourage change. For example, one student tended to pour paint onto the floor of the art therapy room and then smear it. The art therapist had a feeling that it was difficult for him to distinguish between inside and outside. Treatment involved pouring the paint into boxes and containers, which also created an art product. Collecting the paint inside a box helped the student go back to class with a more organized mindset. Discussing the process that he went through with the staff helped them legitimize their negative feelings toward his behavior but also look differently at what could be done to contain the pouring and smearing. Other art therapists commented that with this particular population, work must continue outside the art therapy room and involve multidisciplinary thinking to advance common goals.

CLINICAL ILLUSTRATION

David, 17 years old, is enrolled in a special education school for moderate-functioning students with IDD. He is the eldest child in his family and has two younger siblings. His parents are very invested in helping him and are troubled by his approaching adulthood and finding the right follow-up framework. David has been in music therapy for several years and this year it was decided to transfer him to art therapy as part of an attempt to help him get used to transitions and promote flexibility. In the first sessions, David had a very hard time even entering the art therapy room. The art therapist invited him to join her, but when this failed, she went for a walk with him in the schoolyard. Slowly a connection was made between them and about a month later David agreed to go into the room for the first time.

Inside the art therapy room was a large drawing board hanging on the wall. Next to it was a gouache table: a row of containers each with a separate color and a suitable brush. The art therapist hung a piece of paper on the board and explained to David that he could draw whatever he wanted. She showed him how to work with the gouache table, how to use a different color each time, and how to put each brush back in place. David hesitated. He looked at the gouache and the paper and seemed to not really know what was required of him. The art therapist hung another piece of paper, took a paintbrush with paint, and made a mark on the paper. David looked interested. This ended the first session in the art therapy room.

A week later, when the art therapist went to the classroom, David smiled and agreed to go with her to the art therapy room. There was already a paper on the board in the room. Slowly and hesitantly, he dipped the brush in red, walked toward the paper, and began to draw red circles on it. He looked pleased. When he returned to the gouache table, the art therapist suggested he could change colors and he switched to yellow. He dipped the paint in the container again, went to the paper, and drew more and more yellow circles. Vortices formed on the paper and began to mix with each other. When the paper became cluttered, the art therapist suggested replacing it and hanging up a new, clean sheet of paper. The session continued with more circles on different papers.

In the following months, David went happily to the art therapy room and continued to produce a series of paintings, all colored, and all composed of many circles of various sizes along the length and width of the paper. The art therapist stood next to him, looked at him encouragingly as he continued creating, switched sheets of paper, and most of all enjoyed seeing the extent to which the work made David happy. The classroom educator reported that David waited excitedly for the sessions and returned relaxed from the art therapy room. Some six months later, while making circles, a drop dripped on the bottom of David's paper. He looked with interest at the dot and began to make more. This is how dots entered his paintings. The art therapist excitedly noted that something new had been engendered in his paintings.

David continued to go to the art therapy room for years. The art therapist continued to accompany him in his creative process and whenever something new came up, she admired the novelty, which seems to make David happy too. Alongside the expansion of his pictorial artistic language, there was a softening in his psyche and an expansion of his functions. David began to have a larger behavioral repertoire in the classroom, his social connections multiplied, and he began to engage in organized activities such as trips, and performances outside of school. Toward the age of 21 when graduation and the move to a hostel approached, the art therapist began to prepare David for the separation from treatment as well. She suggested he paint a picture on a very large canvas, that he could take with him to the hostel. David looked excited. He stood in front of the large canvas, adding shapes and colors to it for several weeks from the circles that characterized his first paintings to other styles that he had developed over the years. The painting represented a summary of David's work in art therapy that he could take with him to tell his story.

SUMMARY

Art therapy with students with IDD has a number of specific goals. The first is to encourage the expression of a wide range of emotions even in situations where there are no words to express them. In the process, students can also develop creativity and express it, which also leads to a greater sense of competence. All the interviewees cited the issue of repetition and the need to work on expansion, flexibility, and finding a better balance. When possible, in terms of the level of functioning, students can be helped to move from the concrete to the symbolic and understand the possibility of playful creation that sometimes expresses fantasy. Within art therapy, a meaningful connection is created with an adult that includes acceptance and suspension of judgment, where students can express themselves authentically and know that whatever happens they will be accepted in the art therapy room. For higher functioning students, art therapy can help develop observation, mentalization, awareness of their strengths and weaknesses, how these are presented to others, and how to handle important crossroads in life. For lower-functioning students, art therapists are important mediators, who can help voice clients' experiences and gain a greater understanding of their clients through work in the art therapy room.

The main challenge to art therapists is the slowness of the treatment of clients with IDD. This can lead to frustration and fatigue. Art therapists need a great deal of patience and the ability to recognize and celebrate small changes and assess their significance for these students.

Loneliness in and outside the art therapy room also emerged as a significant hurdle. Some art therapists described their own feelings of rejection of these students when confronted with poor hygiene or extreme situations such as when younger students try to manipulate their environment through deliberately deviant behavior. Finally, some interviewees noted conflictual situations where they feel students are capable of far more independence than acknowledged or authorized by their parents.

Unlike previous chapters in this book, the interventions suggested by the art therapists were divided into two main groups. Some art therapists argued that the nonjudgmental container they provide constitutes a seedbed for the development of creative processes that do not need to be accelerated. These therapists accepted repetitive activities, praised developments verbally, and implemented mirroring to convey their full acceptance. An open studio can facilitate these processes. On the other hand, other art therapists offered a wide range of interventions that they believe can help expand the clients' creative processes. These interventions included offering a specific art material or technique at appropriate moments in treatment. These involved working within diaries through a wide range of art-making techniques or using cell phones as an additional stimulus, as well as group work built around a variety of themes and ways of working. All the art therapists mentioned the need for flexibility to help students, especially the very young or those in transition to enter the art therapy room. In situations of moderate and low functioning, they also suggested the use of alternative supportive communication to help express emotions and choices.

REFERENCES

Ashby, E. (2011). Resourceful, skillful and flexible: Art therapy with people who have severe learning disabilities and challenging behaviour, Chapter 7. In A. Gilroy (Ed.), Art Therapy Research in Practice (pp. 159–180). Peter Lang.

Carrigan, J. (1993). Painting therapy: A Swiss experience for people with mental retardation. American Journal of Art Therapy, 32(2), 53–57.

Ho, R. T., Chan, C. K., Fong, T. C., Lee, P. H., Lum, D. S., & Suen, S. H. (2020). Effects of expressive arts-based interventions on adults with intellectual disabilities: A stratified randomized controlled trial. Frontiers in Psychology, 11, 1286.

Lett, C. (2005). Increasing expression in an adult male with Down syndrome and moderate mental retardation. Ursuline College.

Trzaska, J. D. (2012). The use of a group mural project to increase self-esteem in high-functioning, cognitively disabled adults. *The Arts in Psychotherapy, 39*(5), 436–442.

White, I., Bull, S., & Beavis, M. (2009). Isobel's images – One woman's experience of art therapy. *British Journal of Learning Disabilities, 37*(2), 103–109.

BRIEF BIOGRAPHIES OF THE ART THERAPISTS WHO CONTRIBUTED TO THIS CHAPTER

Tami Avraham, art therapist (M.A.) and supervisor, has worked for 12 years as an art therapist in a special education school for students with IDD.

Irit Belity, art therapist (M.A.) and supervisor, lecturer at the School of Creative Arts Therapies at the University of Haifa, has worked for 21 years as an art therapist, including 6 years as an art therapist in a special education school for students with IDD.

Yael Domany, art therapist (M.A.) and supervisor, lecturer at the School of Creative Arts Therapies at the University of Haifa, has worked for 21 years as an art therapist, including 12 years as an art therapist for students and adults with IDD.

Tal Goffer, art therapist (M.A.) and psychotherapist, has worked for nine years as an art therapist in the education system, including six years as an art therapist for students with IDD.

Lilach Herzog, art therapist and educational counselor (M.A.), has worked for 21 years as an art therapist in the education system, including 15 years as an art therapist for children with IDD in a special education kindergarten and a special education school for students with IDD.

Dan Polak, art therapist (Ph.D.) and supervisor, lecturer at the ASA – Ono Academic College, has worked for 25 years as an art therapist and sexual therapist including 15 years as an art therapist in a special education school for students with IDD.

Ronny Seri, art therapist (M.A.), has worked for 15 years as an art therapist, including 12 years as an art therapist in a special education school for students with IDD.

Six

INTRODUCTION

Children with compromised social and emotional health are at considerable risk. Psychological problems have been shown to have a negative impact on children's ability to fulfill their educational and developmental potential. The onset of emotional and behavioral disorders can often be traced back to the school years, making this a crucial population to target (Cortina & Fazel, 2015).

The art therapists characterized students with behavioral disorders in the special education system as children who come close to dropping out of school, whom the education system wants to give one last chance. Frequently these students have lost all confidence in the system in general and in authority figures in particular as a result of conflicts and disappointments. They are usually in a state of despair. Some cope with undiagnosed and untreated conditions such as attention-deficit/ hyperactivity disorder (ADD/ADHD), exacerbated by a later behavioral disorder. Some have gone through traumatic experiences or come from difficult home environments. This may place them on a victim-aggressor, controlling-dominating continuum. One art therapist considered that they are in fact survivors who have learned that violence and aggression constitute their only way of dealing with a world they feel is constantly attacking them. The interviewees who work in special schools for students with behavioral disorders felt that their main goal was to enable these students to return to regular schools after three to four years of treatment, although this objective is not always achieved.

One art therapist said that over the years she has identified two major groups of students with behavioral disorders in special education. One group is composed of students who are constantly exploding, harassing, losing control, and getting into trouble. The second group

DOI: 10.4324/9781003156918-6

is composed of very sensitive, anxious, willing students, who do not really grasp why they were assigned to this school. However, when they do explode, they are in maximal survival mode, as though fighting for their lives.

Conducting a successful art therapy group for children with emotional and behavioral disorders is extremely challenging since these students tend to resist the rules, limits, and boundaries of a group setting. The therapist must learn to maintain the appropriate balance between structure and flexibility within the therapeutic framework to foster each child's feelings of security, safety, and containment and to maximize the child's creativity and therapeutic growth (Perkins, 2007). A study that analyzed teachers' ratings of the effects of arts therapy-related experiences on the behavior of children exposed to abuse and poverty indicated that they displayed fewer externalized behavioral problems (aggressive and delinquent behavior) as a result of therapy (Kim & Kim, 2014).

THE THERAPEUTIC GOALS OF ART THERAPY

The main goal of art therapy for this population is to restore these students' trust in people and to foster their belief that their art therapist is on their side, that difficult things can be expressed through artwork or verbally, and that they can be contained in the art therapy room. One interviewee emphasized that in special education schools for students with behavioral disorders, each student is typically given an individual hour of therapy because each of them needs an intimate and protected place to begin to deal with the numerous difficulties they face. Another art therapist emphasized that it is precisely these students who most need to be in psychotherapy/arts therapy because their most fundamental needs have not been met. At the same time, the characteristics of therapy including the intimate space, the safe place, the symbolic space, and the permission to be a child, be playful, and communicate freely are threatening to them. The very fact of remaining with an adult in the art therapy room is not self-evident and gaining trust can take months. One of the art therapists emphasized that every step these students take is experienced as a mountain that needs to be climbed and they must feel that the effort will bear fruit. She constantly reminds herself of her difficult first years as a novice art therapist to avoid dulling her senses, in order to be attuned and contain the initial feelings of new students to the school.

Another key goal is to promote these students' ability to communicate. These students often feel humiliated or defeated when they need help. The goal is to learn that a need or difficulty can be expressed and answered, and that needs do not need to be expressed solely by acting out. To help the students express their feelings and desires to the staff as well, the therapists work closely with the educational staff. Because these students' initial relationship was often very damaged and their communication patterns are rigid, they often misinterpret situations, which leads them to misjudge social interactions. Thus, another goal of art therapy is related to interactions with others.

The art therapists emphasized the importance of enabling these students to regain control over their lives. This begins within the art therapy room and extends later to the world outside. This includes teaching students to listen to their bodies and creating an inner monitor or guardrail that warns them whenever they are about to lose control. Treatment also addresses the issues that cause the client to explode and lose control. This can be done in collaboration with the educational staff. For example, if the most suitable coping pattern for a particular student is to step outside the classroom for a few minutes, the staff is encouraged to accept this behavior.

A number of art therapists emphasized that the goals of art therapy are heavily dependent on the students' progression. Since students are typically enrolled in a special school for a number of years, the primary goal when they arrive is to enable them to adapt to the new framework. This includes building trust, gaining confidence, strengthening their sense of competence, and raising hope. One art therapist noted that art therapy is the only subject in school that is not obligatory so it needs to be presented to the students in a way that will encourage them to remain in therapy. When students are about to return to the regular education system or will soon graduate, the goal is to help them integrate into their next academic framework or enter real life, sometimes gradually. In between, the emphasis is on building self-worth and a more positive self-image and on developing mental flexibility which involves grasping that at any given time there are different ways of responding and that retaliation is not always the only or most successful alternative. Since many students are also diagnosed with oppositional defiant disorder (ODD), they can lock quickly into one response mode and need to be helped to see that there are other choices open to them.

CHALLENGES

All the art therapists described instances when it was very difficult to contain these students. These students are characterized by bursts of aggression, violence, chaos, and a strong sense of helplessness. Sometimes students need to be physically separated, which is physically and emotionally draining. The art therapists described schools in which there was constant running, pushing, shouting, and the constant pressure to be on the alert to respond when someone exploded. Sometimes students cry or need to be held because they may explode and hurt themselves or others. Some therapists said that they had never dealt with this population before and that at times the experience was overwhelming. One interviewee said that at first, even reading the students' files was difficult, since their experiences were so devastating. The art therapists described their intense feelings of compassion for the students, and their enormous anger at their parents for abandoning, hurting, or just not being there for them.

One art therapist said that containing despair was his major stumbling block. These desperate children, who often come from broken homes, have become a punching bag for years in their homes and in the school system. This despair is further exacerbated by the fact that there is no parental holding. Despair tends to manifest initially as violent behavior, which is why these students were transferred to the special school. Teamwork is needed to contain this despair. However, this art therapist noted that the hard part is the depressive symptomatology that emerges later.

Another difficulty that was mentioned involves situations where a student engages in very regressive behavior in the art therapy room, sometimes bordering on disintegration. These moments can be very frightening, when the art therapist needs to help the student calm down and return to class, sometimes quite quickly when another student is already waiting at the door.

One art therapist described the enormous difficulty of disclosing difficult information revealed by students, some of which require reporting. For instance, one student told his art therapist that he had a knife in his bag; another student described torturing animals. These situations require a careful, gentle approach to avoid damaging the therapeutic alliance. Even after a strong therapeutic relationship has been established, students may also commit a significant offense that results in their expulsion from school, thus leaving the therapist feeling very helpless.

In a similar context, it is also important for the art therapist to differentiate between the rehearsal of violent impulses and their sublimation in adolescent imagery. Rehearsal has an element of conscious awareness and planning, whereas sublimation is typically an unconscious process (Phillips, 2003). Art can be a mode of expression where the adolescent plans and/or rehearses violence. Violent images may depict something the adolescent is considering putting into action. This can be difficult to judge and requires an excellent rapport as well as strong clinical skills and experience. In particular, an awareness of the source of the imagery can help differentiate between rehearsal and sublimation (Phillips, 2003).

Finding a suitable art therapy room within the educational framework also poses a challenge for therapeutic work with these students. Given their difficulties deciding to go and to stay in the art therapy room, a secluded, quiet room where therapist and client are not disturbed by events at school is a must. In addition, the room should include an area or cupboard where art materials that are less suitable at the moment for a particular student can be locked away. The exposure of all the art materials can lead to complete destruction. To conclude this section, one of the art therapists addressed the difficulty of students persevering with a creative work overtime. Both engaging in the work and sticking with it is a challenge for many students.

INTERVENTION TECHNIQUES AND DEDICATED WORKING MODELS

The art therapist's positioning in the case of aggressive behavior

One of the most interesting aspects that emerged from the interviews was the art therapist's positioning in cases of aggressive behavior. Although at first it seemed to me that this issue might be related to differences between a dynamic and a CBT (cognitive behavioral therapy) theoretical approach, the interviewees' comments made it clear that this was not necessarily the case. Some art therapists want to know what is happening to their clients outside the art therapy room and incorporate this information into the therapeutic session in a variety of ways. In their view, precisely because they work within the education system, this connection is required. In contrast, other art therapists argued that they do not have to know and even if they do know, they will not relate to aggressive behavior outside the art therapy room themselves, unless the client raises it. They feel that because they work in a team where the teachers contain the behavioral issues, they can actually allow the student to be in a therapeutic bubble, containing only what s/he wishes to include. Some argued that staff members understood and supported this choice, while others noted that this attitude led to criticism from staff members.

A dialectic model for art therapy (Nissimov-Nahum, 2008, 2021)

Nissimov-Nahum's model addresses the importance of cooperation between major players in the child's life and ways of dealing with aggressive behavior. It puts forward three areas of intervention and hypothesizes that the effects of all three concurrently are essential to the success of treatment. The most important area is the interpersonal space, the relationship between the art therapist and the student. Another space for action is the systemic space, where the art therapist attempts to make meaningful contact with the parents and the student's educators, in order to expand the influence of the treatment on the client's life. This space also includes providing supervision to the school staff on how to work with the student. Finally, the personal space enables the art therapist to examine his/her personal experiences in depth. Within each of these spaces, the art therapist works according to two principles. The first is the creation of a space of acceptance, both as a response to the needs of the client and his/her environment and as a response to the inner needs of the art therapist. The second, seemingly contradictory principle, is a commitment to change. These two principles of acceptance and change are dialectically related to each other and reinforce each other. Acceptance encourages change, since when clients feel accepted, they may let go of destructive parts of themselves and believe in change. On the other hand, with the intention of change, clients understand that acceptance does not condone aggressive behavior.

Boundaries vs. flexibility

All the art therapists emphasized the importance of setting boundaries for treatment in the art therapy room. The session takes place on a set day, at a set time and place. Some also noted that certain behaviors cannot be tolerated in the art therapy room and that there are cases where the session is terminated immediately even in the middle (e.g., a student lighting a cigarette in the room). These boundaries can be more contained or looser than the boundaries typically found in the educational system, but the art therapy room is still a place that enforces its own rules.

On the other hand, some art therapists reported tailoring the therapeutic setting to each client. This setting is designed to help students be treated in a way that suits them best. One interviewee said that sometimes the sessions take place outside because it seems to be the right thing for a particular student. For example, he described working for a long period of a time with a student at the pool table. It started as an attempt to recruit the student for art therapy and continued through joint play and an attempt to work on inhibition, power regulation, and law enforcement. He had sessions with another student at football games, which were aimed at helping him deal with social anxiety.

A dynamic approach to art therapy

The art therapists primarily applied two major theoretical approaches. The primary one was the dynamic approach, which is not always easy to implement within an educational framework. One art therapist described how she only barely manages to maintain her dynamic attitude toward students. She tries not to allow external events to affect the art therapy room bubble and not to allow content from the art therapy room to leak out into daily life at school. She felt that it was precisely these students who had experienced so much intrusion from the environment, who needed to feel they were in a clean dynamic container, with no outside intervention. This also meant that she refused to be involved in the students' behavioral program, tried to keep the atmosphere as open and welcoming as possible in the art therapy room, and allowed the students a wide range of experiences using the art materials. The better she knew the students and the better they were contained by the educational staff, the more confident she felt and was able to allow the students a wide choice of art materials. Most students were attracted by printed magazines and newspapers that could be flipped through and sometimes used to create a collage, clay that could be hit and sometimes even led to a finished product (like a mask in a mold), plaster that could be molded and painted, woodwork including wood carving, work with pulp and color mixes, work with cartons and boxes, work on large sheets of paper, work in a sandbox. These relatively familiar materials can give the student an experience of success even though it also results in many unfinished works. Any work that could be continued over a number of sessions was a great achievement. Sometimes the transition between art materials was meaningful, for instance, moving from hard materials such as wood to soft materials such as yarn and fabric. The art therapist also described how important it was to the students that she brought art materials to the art therapy room that they wanted but were not available. In this way, she showed that she was thinking about them even beyond the therapeutic hour. The creative work mostly involved destruction, which was repeated and included cutting, throwing, scattering, tearing, etc. Then, at times, students began gluing with hot glue or using nails or even sewing or fusing fragments together. In addition, much of the work was inside and with containers such as boxes or bowls or folders that contained pieces of work and the whole. The discourse that accompanied the creative work often dealt with the clients' projections about events in their lives and how their vulnerability turned into splits, and the sense that the world was against them.

Another art therapist who works according to the dynamic approach said that the cupboard in the art therapy room contains a variety of art materials, but that she only allows students to open it, take out materials and then close the door, so that in the event of an outburst of rage, there will not be too much destruction in the room. She tries very hard to avoid flooding with too many stimuli. The art materials help create a container for anger and aggression and allow them to be regulated. This includes objects that enable destruction, breakage, disassembly and assembly, regressive materials, woodworking materials for sawing, construction and deconstruction, throwing clay for pottery-making, construction and dismantling of cartons, making weapons and swords, throwing and catching balls, soft materials (a loom, sewing, knitting) where there was something in the repetitiveness and softness that really attracted the students, and sandbox work where they can work and then efface it. She explicitly wondered whether children with such primary vulnerabilities can actually be helped by CBT, or whether the dynamic approach is the best choice since the defense mechanisms the students use are still very primitive, such as projection and split.

Cognitive behavioral therapy (CBT) for art therapy

Other art therapists described how they incorporated CBT principles into art therapy. One said she did so primarily when students were engaged in problematic behavior. Information about these incidents can come from the student him/herself or from the staff members which she then shares with the student. She asks the students to describe what happened, how s/he felt, and they analyze the event together. She also suggested that the students describe it in art and present it visually. Another art therapist incorporates elements of planning and flexible thinking within the creative process by talking with the student about what s/he wants to build and the ways it can be done. Later, this form of thinking can be extended to other aspects of life as a way of looking at cause and effect. In addition, he tries to find a way to evaluate the baseline level of students' behavior to be able to gauge changes. Since it is difficult for students to do this on their own, and at home there is often no one to help them, he often asks the teaching staff to help monitor evolutions in behavior. One art therapist uses the class setting to help students cope better. For example, she sometimes prepares a box for clients that contains items that can remind them of behavioral exercises for coping that they have practiced together, and she instructs the teacher to refer these students to the box in moments of crisis and outbursts.

Structure of the therapeutic session

Several art therapists described how they structure the therapeutic session by dividing it into several parts. For example, at the beginning of the session, there can be structured work on emotions with an emotions board to let the student express current feelings. Then, she offers students to take part in physical activities such as jumping on a trampoline, playing ball, hitting a punching bag, etc. After the physical activity, the students are invited to engage in artwork. In schools that have a number of art therapy rooms, the therapist can select the setting that best corresponds to the student. Some of the interviewees also described the gradual evolution in the number of different art materials. Markers and work with print media are suggested first and students only work with more regressive materials later, as the therapeutic alliance strengthens. The parameters dictating which art materials to present in each session are guided by the students' overall state, their state on a given day, the extent of familiarity with their work with art materials, and the developmental stage. One therapist also inserts predefined components into the creative work such as building a circle of emotions where students choose a color for each emotion and can draw with those colors.

Working on sensory, emotional, and behavioral regulation using art materials

Some art therapists described artwork with materials that can be manipulated without necessarily turning them into a product, such as clay, plasticine, dough, and kinetic sand. The very act of holding, kneading, and touching helps regulation. Other art therapists mentioned tools and materials that they would restrict or not give to students. For example, one art therapist who works with wood said she would allow students to work with a hammer and nails and a saw, but not with more dangerous tools. She pays close attention when students use knives for slicing. Art therapists who work with this population tend to lock up Japanese knives, scissors, sharpened pencils, or anything else that could cause injury.

Spinning plates

Einat Arad described a technique she developed while working with a class of children with behavioral problems that primarily included excessive movement.

> The challenge was to turn the scattered, flooding movement into growth that is positive, focused and reserved. The children's and staff's movements evoked an association of rotational movement, and it occurred to me to develop work with colors on a rotating plate.

The device is a battery-driven motor connected to a wooden box that spins a plastic plate. When the motor is switched on, the plate rotates, and the student draws on it with markers, watercolors, or gouache. Circles and spirals are created on the plate that evokes a sense of surprise and success and increases motivation. This technique can help develop focus, concentration, and emotional regulation, and has attracted considerable attention (for a video, see www.earad.co.il).

Working with clients' violent imagery

When confronted with clients' violent imagery, art therapists must be willing to plunge into the darker side of life to explore these adolescents' relationship to violence. Exploring their own fantasies, fears, and imagery is crucial to understanding the meanings the adolescents ascribe to their art expressions. A number of guidelines can help effectively tap their creative and healing potential without reinforcing or dismissing violent content. These include efforts to (1) Avoid reacting to violent imagery with disgust, fear, or extreme shock. (2) Allow, support, and at times, even encourage the expression of strong affect, which can include anger, aggression, or violence, in adolescent art. (3) Explore the meaning of the work with the adolescent. (4) Develop and encourage creative expression overall, not just the violent content. (5) Value the skill evidenced even when not valuing the content of the art and communicate this very clearly and consistently. (6) Look for creative alternatives for the expression of violent imagery and/or associated feelings (Phillips, 2003).

Group-class art therapy model

Many art therapists also provide group-class art therapy. Most noted that they try not to work individually with students while in a group setting, so that the students do not feel obligated to "share" the therapist with others during group work. One of the art therapists emphasized that these students' level of trust is extremely fragile, and how easily the therapeutic alliance can fissure within the group space. By contrast, another art therapist said she prefers to take individual clients from the class she works with as a group, as her ability to see students within the group class, including in interactions with other students, allows her to continue working individually on content that also came up in the group setting.

In all the cases described, the educator and assistant are also present in the group class art therapy sessions. One interviewee emphasized that the educator and assistant actually constitute the parenting model of the class and the art therapist introduces the emotional content into this space. One of the goals of group-class art therapy is to incorporate communication content so that it becomes a place where words can be spoken and not just acted out. In most cases, after each session, an hour is devoted to co-processing the experience, both verbally and through art (so that the educator and assistant can experience the techniques on themselves as well). The role of the educator and assistant varies depending on the art therapist's orientation. Sometimes they are actually invited to participate in the group and engage in a form of modeling for the students but at other times they are mainly responsible for containment and disciplinary issues.

One art therapist described how working in this format forces her to adapt her creativity to the current class mood. Group-class art therapy is usually structured. It begins with an opening ceremony with clear rules of group behavior where the students say how they feel. Sometimes group participants hand each other a speech stick, which only allows the person holding it to talk. Sometimes there is a sign reminding students to be quiet. The staff members can be asked to sit in different locations in the class and can contribute through their presence. Sometimes the group develops gradually, in that students first work individually, then in pairs, then in small groups, and only at the end if behaviorally feasible the whole class together. One of the interviewees described how she chooses an annual topic for the group each time. For example, for the transition to junior high, a theme could be "the journey to junior high". The students determine the strengths that they have and strengths that they would like to acquire over the course of the year. They can make a backpack or suitcase at the beginning of the year where they collect the works they do during the year. The activities should be attractive to the students and involve considerable creativity (e.g., taking pictures in the school yard that represent different aspects of this journey). Another art therapist described providing a common substrate on which the group could create together, but where the students only decide on the theme after discussing it together. Yet another art therapist noted that the exercises she brought were very measured and structured, and that their main purpose was to expand the students' play ability.

In another school, one interviewee indicated that the group work is usually guided by a topic and can take place in the classroom setting or with combined classes. For example, she described a year in which the staff decided to form a group for new students because they felt there was a real need. As part of the group work, the rules and regulations were explained, and the students talked about how best to fit in. It was also a place to share the difficult feelings of adaptation to a new school. In another instance, they formed a group whose theme was making connections for students who seemed to need it.

THE MEANING OF ART

Waller (2006) suggested that art made in the safe confines of the art therapy room may enable a child to explore and express feelings that cannot easily be put into words. Instead of acting out "difficult" feelings, the child puts them into an object. It can then be shared with the art therapist. The art can act as a "container" for powerful emotions and as a means of communication between child and art therapist. The interviewees stressed that art is first and foremost a means of expression for these students, a way of expressing their inner world which is often very flooded. Beyond expression, the act of making art itself can also have a calming influence.

One art therapist considered that art is also a release from the burden of the spoken word. The spoken word requires a great deal of effort from these students and is far removed from an authentic expression of the self. He stressed that these students experience the most criticism for their verbal outbursts so that being freed of the obligation to use words can help them to express feelings. This is also why words sometimes emerge at a much later stage in therapy. Art can also confer a sense of competence, in particular since these students who have experienced multiple frustrations in their lives have not had the opportunity to reveal their abilities. The possibility of doing so concretely becomes a source of power.

COLLABORATIVE INTERVENTIONS INVOLVING PARENTS AND STAFF MEMBERS

Working with parents

Working with parents is crucial. One art therapist stated she took concerted steps to maintain a connection, whether face to face or over the phone. Parental contact enables the art therapist to mediate the students' needs and desires to their parents. All the interviewees noted that working with parents is highly complex, since they are often not interested in establishing a relationship with the art therapist, perhaps because of their complex familial issues.

Some schools organize art therapy groups for parents of students with behavioral disorders. The purpose of these sessions is to make it clear to parents that they are not alone, and that other parents face similar difficulties. The group engages in activities to foster learning how to deal with their children more effectively, especially in CBT orientations. The interventions are both verbal and through art. For example, parents can be given a prompt such as "Draw yourself and your child in two colors on the page". The artwork can help clarify the components of the relationship. Despite interest on the part of the staff to facilitate such groups, the art therapists who lead these groups noted that parents rarely attended or came back for further sessions. By contrast, one art therapist led a successful Zoom group to support parents during the pandemic.

Working with staff members

Almost all of the art therapists interviewed for this chapter considered that they formed a team with the staff and that they worked as a family. They praised the very special people who dedicate themselves to working with these students and do so wholeheartedly. For many of them, this is what helps them to survive in the very complex situations they experience.

One interviewee described teamwork in a class of students with behavioral disorders integrated in a regular school. The art therapists mediated the students' difficulties to the school staff to help them deal with classroom challenges. The same therapist also described joint work by the educational–therapeutic staff in a behavioral program tailored to each student. At the end of each lesson, each student is evaluated as to whether his or her behavioral goals were met. Progress is indicated by changing the color of the goal sheet displayed in class so that anyone entering the classroom can see the changes.

Another art therapist noted that students are highly sensitive to the relationship between the art therapist and the educational staff which if interpreted negatively can undermine the therapeutic relationship.

Her solution is to only contact the teachers in the teachers' room, where students are not allowed. On the other hand, another art therapist emphasized how important it is not to create splits. That is, if she sees a difficult event involving one of her clients in school, she tells the student that she saw it, to avoid contributing to a situation where the difficulties are split and do not enter the art therapy room. In other cases, the educational staff members sometimes call the art therapist when they see that one of the students is on the verge of an explosion and they think s/he might be able to help him/her. Sometimes the therapist turns to staff members when s/he identifies something in the session that should be followed or addressed.

The art therapists emphasized the need for support, assistance, and containment from the educational framework. One art therapist described the efforts made by the school principal to make sure that the staff was contained before the start of the year. The teachers and assistants all received support and guidance from the art therapist when working in the group-class model. The arts therapists themselves received support through supervision.

CLINICAL ILLUSTRATION

Yossi was sent to a special school for behavioral disorders when he was 15. His mother had died five years previously and his father was in and out of psychiatric hospitals. In recent years, he had lived in a number of foster homes without finding a successful solution for him. His behavioral problems became more frequent as was his feeling of desperation that he had nothing to live for. The art therapist who read his file immediately realized that most of all Yossi needed confidence and a rebuilding of his trust in human beings.

In the first month, the staff at the school observed Yossi from a distance to determine what he liked and what made him angry, who he engaged with, and what situations tended to trigger aggressive behavior. It was not an easy start. Yossi overturned tables in the classroom and kicked angrily when he did not get what he wanted. When offered to go to a weekly session with the art therapist, he refused and claimed that everyone at the school was being paid to be with him and they were not acting in his best interests. The art therapist continued searching for a way to get him to go to the art therapy room and asked his educator what he liked to do. It turned out that there was one board game in the class called Taki that he really liked and was willing to play with anyone.

One day, the art therapist approached the school principal and asked her to tell Yossi that the staff had decided to allow him one hour a week to play Taki with one of the staff members. The staff member chosen was of course the art therapist. Yossi was happy to hear about the new arrangement. At first, the sessions took place in a playroom. Yossi was very suspicious, put his hoodie over his head and barely looked up from the game, but kept coming back week after week. At first, he did not talk at all except to keep the game going. Then, little by little, the art therapist tentatively asked him how he was or how he was doing during class or during the breaks. At the same time, outbursts of rage continued to occur when Yossi was required to do something, and his functioning remained poor.

After several months of play, when from time to time the art therapist was able to see Yossi's eyes or extract a sentence or two from him, she asked whether he would like to see the art therapy room. Yossi entered hesitantly and looked at the art materials in the cupboard. He took out a piece of plasticine and began to knead it. Then, he walked toward the window and looked out. Finally, he placed the plasticine on the table and left the room without saying a word.

A week later he was waiting for the art therapist at the art therapy door for his session. They went in together and he walked over to a bowl filled with kinetic sand. He touched it, picked up some sand and watched it glide between his fingers, and again sank his hand deep into the sand. The art therapist stood next to him and after a few minutes of play, showed him how to photograph hands collecting the sand and scattering it on top of the container in slow motion. Yossi agreed and during the next hour they photographed hands and sand together.

This is how a durable connection between Yossi and the art therapist slowly began to form, which extended for years to come. Inside the art therapy room, he slowly began to work, first in sand and plaster and later also in gouache. Yossi worked on masks for a long time, making frightening black and red masks week after week that began to express the horror and loneliness he had experienced in his life in his own way. It was almost wordless therapy, with a great deal of doing, and imagery. It helped Yossi tell the art therapist his story. At the same time, his behavior improved, and his tantrums diminished.

Toward the age of 18, Yossi started to prepare for graduation. In treatment, the art therapist gently tried to say something about life after school. They discussed possibilities for Yossi in the post-school reality. During the last session, the art therapist was very emotional since he had touched her heart. She wrote him a long letter describing their journey together. In simple sentences, she described the miraculous process he had gone through. Yossi did not open the letter during the session and said goodbye succinctly, which frustrated the art therapist. A year later he wrote to her on WhatsApp: "Since we said goodbye, there has not been a day that I have not read the letter you wrote to me. It has helped me continue my life after school".

SUMMARY

The art therapists interviewed here who work with students with behavioral disorders in special classes within a regular school and in special schools all underscored a number of goals for art therapy with these students. The prime goal of treatment is to restore these students' trust in people in general, while establishing a nurturing connection with the art therapist. Art therapy can help develop these students' communication skills so that they feel they can talk about all kinds of things and that there are people who are willing to listen to them. They do not have to act out in response to internal and external stimuli. Art therapy can help students regain control over their lives, initially through the art materials in the art therapy room and later through building an inner guardrail, which will help them in cases of loss of control. Finally, the art therapists emphasized that the goals must be tailored to the student's stage which ranges from adapting to the school framework, separation, and the transition to another framework or back to the community.

The main difficulty in working with these students is containing them physically and emotionally. The art therapists described their ceremonies of transition and preparation before going to work and how important it is for them to be assisted by a supportive staff and receive appropriate supervision. Some of the students' life stories are unbearable and they are required to be a container for their despair and accompany them even in very regressive and broken situations. Very difficult content can arise both verbally and in art. This content can lead to concerns as to whether to disclose, since the students' aggressive behavior can constitute a risk for themselves and for the school environment. Finding an appropriate art therapy room is crucial to be able to contain this content in full confidentiality and trust.

The art therapists found it difficult to determine how much of these students' violent and aggressive reality should enter the art therapy room. Some felt that it could not be ignored and that their job was to connect the outside world with the inner world of the students. Others felt that they could only handle a bubble containing what the student decided to include. Some mentioned the dialectical model which deals with multi-system work and the constant connection between acceptance and commitment to change. Most addressed their theoretical approach, where some art therapists considered that only dynamic work was appropriate for these students; others also incorporated aspects of CBT. All concurred that along with defined time limits, there is also a need for a great deal of flexibility to devise the most effective way to reach out to each client. The art materials contribute to sensory, emotional, and behavioral regulation, and each art therapist found a way to structure the therapeutic session to suit each client. Most also worked in the class-group settings where relationships could be observed, and steps taken to help these students find better ways to connect with others.

REFERENCES

Cortina, M. A., & Fazel, M. (2015). The art room: An evaluation of a targeted school-based group intervention for students with emotional and behavioural difficulties. The Arts in Psychotherapy, 42, 35–40.

Kim, J., & Kim, K. (2014). Behavioral and musical characteristics of the children who are exposed to child maltreatment and poverty in South Korea: A survey. Child Abuse & Neglect, 38(6), 1023–1032.

Nissimov-Nahum, E. (2008). A model for art therapy in educational settings with children who behave aggressively. The Arts in Psychotherapy, 35(5), 341–348.

Nissimov-Nahum, E. (2021). A dialectic model for art therapy with students who behave aggressively. In D. Regev & S. Snir (Eds.), Integrating arts therapies into education (pp. 128–146). Routledge.

Perkins, S. (2007). Creating containment and facilitating freedom: Group art therapy with children with emotional and behavioural disorders (Doctoral dissertation, Concordia University).

Phillips, J. (2003). Working with adolescents' violent imagery. In C.A., Malchiodi, Handbook of Art Therapy (pp. 229–238). Guilford Press.

Waller, D. (2006). Art therapy for children: How it leads to change. Clinical Child Psychology and Psychiatry, 11(2), 271–282.

BRIEF BIOGRAPHIES OF THE ART THERAPISTS WHO CONTRIBUTED TO THIS CHAPTER

Einat Arad, art therapist (M.A.) and supervisor, has worked for 18 years as an art therapist in the education system, including 12 years as an art therapist for children with behavioral disorders.

Hanna Ekshtein-Rain, art therapist (M.A.) and supervisor, has worked for 19 years as an art therapist, including 10 years in a special education school for students with behavioral disorders.

Dror Kaufman, art therapist (M.A.) and supervisor, has worked for 21 years in a special education school for students with behavioral disorders including 11 years as an art therapist.

Revital Turiski, art therapist (M.A.) and supervisor, has worked for 12 years as an art therapist in the education system, including 9 years in a special education school for students with behavioral disorders.

Anat Yefet, art therapist (M.A.) and supervisor, has worked for eight years as an art therapist in the education system with students with behavioral disorders.

Seven

INTRODUCTION

Many children are hospitalized for varying lengths of time for a variety of medical conditions including illness and accidents. The Ministry of Education in Israel provides a solution for these children through schools that are located in the hospital. These schools also offer arts therapies. The setting for these therapeutic sessions varies. Sometimes it involves working in regular art therapy rooms, while in others it involves working at the client's bedside in the ward where medical equipment, other patients, and the medical staff can be present during the session with the client. The duration of treatment also varies and ranges from single sessions to prolonged treatment for children with chronic diseases. Sometimes a therapeutic session has to be halted for a medical procedure and resumes at a later point in time (Weinfeld-Yehoudayan, 2013). One of the art therapists noted that the referral process is also different in hospitals because art therapists approach potential clients and suggest treatment, so that a major part of the process involves "courting" clients.

This chapter reflects the contributions of art therapists who work in a variety of hospital settings. Some work with children who are in the hospital for short periods of time such as in internal or surgical wards, whereas others work with children who are in the hospital for longer stays such as in the cardiac or oncology wards. Finally, one of the art therapists also works in a rehabilitation hospital, where the setting is again different. I will try to give space and voice to this variety of approaches and possibilities.

Art therapists have a long tradition of working in medical settings. Studies support the usefulness of art therapy in medical settings and have reported associations between art, healing, and public health measures (Metzl et al., 2016; Wigham et al., 2020). Clapp et al. (2019) conducted a systematic review of the benefits of art therapy

DOI: 10.4324/9781003156918-7

in helping children and teens adapt to situations of ill health. Twelve studies (with patients ranging in age from 2 to 19, with various medical conditions) were included. Ten studies reported significant improvements concerning at least one outcome, with an overall inconclusive trend toward effectiveness. Metzl et al. (2016) suggested based on their study that art therapy services should be offered when pain levels are lower, and the client is able to physically and mentally engage in the process. When clients are in a great deal of pain, medical art therapists should consider creating more "passive" art therapy interventions (such as viewing and talking about art, making art for the client or with the client).

Research indicates that children and adolescents with chronic medical problems make more use of health care services and have greater problems with school attendance and their schoolwork. They also experience more psychological maladjustment and/or issues with mental health. There is a wide range of art programs for sick children. For example, Art for Life is a community of arts mentorship program connecting 25 sick children to volunteer artist-mentors for five months each year. The Art for Life program is structured and facilitated by creative arts therapists who recruit community artist-mentors, match them to these students and then provide the therapeutic foundation for one-on-one mentoring relationships. Structured interviews with some of the participants (children, parents, and staff) underscored the importance of these mentorship relationships, which resulted in an increase in students' self-esteem, enhanced family bonds, and the development of new coping skills (Reed et al., 2015). Stafstrom et al. (2012) found that art therapy focus groups can provide a safe, nurturing environment for children and adolescents with epilepsy to explore and discuss their disorder with similarly affected peers, and hence allow for the development of strong interpersonal bonds and better long-term psychosocial functioning.

Several overviews have dealt with art therapy for children with cancer (e.g., Aguilar, 2017; Raybin & Krajicek, 2020). The Aguilar (2017) integrative literature review examined the effectiveness of art therapy for children with cancer. They identified seven studies that met the inclusion criteria for qualitative and quantitative studies. The results suggested that art therapy, in the form of drawing interventions, improved communication with family members and providers, served as a way to express feelings, helped the children to develop effective coping skills, and reduced the negative effects of the treatment (Aguilar, 2017; Kaimal et al., 2019). Favara-Scacco et al. (2001) reported on the impact of providing art therapy to children with leukemia. The main goal was to reduce anxiety and fear during painful interventions as well as prolonged emotional distress. They found that children provided with art therapy as of their first hospitalization exhibited collaborative behavior. They or their parents asked for art therapy when the intervention had to be repeated. The parents declared themselves better able to manage the painful procedures when art therapy was offered. Stinley et al. (2015) explored the feasibility of implementing a fast-acting mandala intervention to reduce physical pain and psychological anxiety experienced during needle insertions. The results indicated that physiological stress behaviors were significantly reduced, and psychological anxiety decreased significantly in the treatment group. These findings support the use of mandalas created on an iPad with pediatric patients undergoing acute pain procedures. Finally, Councill and Ramsey (2019) described a patient and his family who engaged in art therapy over the course of 18 months as an integrated, palliative component of treatment. Art therapy helped this patient and his family navigate four distinct phases of care, from diagnosis to end of life, in response to the family's changing needs. Communicating directly and symbolically at the end of the child's life allowed the family to create a lasting legacy.

THE THERAPEUTIC GOALS OF ART THERAPY

Children in the hospital must undergo a variety of invasive tests and procedures. This elicits an intense feeling of lack of control. Art therapy can encourage the expression of these difficult experiences and give these children a certain sense of control through the choice of creative materials, techniques, and ways of working. The choice of materials, artistic endeavors, and the active nature of the work such as cutting, arranging, designing, pasting, and creating something tangible allows these children to experience themselves as active and capable creators, as opposed to the difficult feeling of being victims of their disease or passive, helpless patients. Thus, children in the hospital who can create, express an active rather than a passive attitude, which can be communicative and undefeated. Often the need for control is also reflected in clients' decisions when and if they go to the art therapy room, when the session will begin, and when it will end. The role of the art therapist is to engage in courtship, establish a negotiation while containing and understanding the sensitivity and needs of the sick child to be in control.

Sometimes the very act of being creative helps to put the pain aside for a time and focus on something else. In addition, since art enables greater expression of difficult experiences, children's stress levels decrease and their cooperation with the medical staff increases (Malchiodi, 2013; Weinfeld-Yehoudayan, 2013). One of the art therapists described how even in cases of a single session she tries to focus on the clients' situation, give meaning to what is happening to them and sometimes also encourage them to talk to the medical staff to get more information. Another therapist said that in the hospital where she works, the staff tries to integrate art therapists as soon as children are admitted to the emergency room, to reduce the trauma they experience by being in a medical framework.

Art therapy is also part of the processing of trauma and loss as well as learning to cope with a variety of diseases and injuries. Children are hospitalized for many different types of trauma – from illness to accidents. Sometimes, there is a loss of a particular function or an organ and the realization that their lives are going to change entirely. Art therapy can begin to allow this content to be reconstructed and processed, first through the creative work and later also through words. The artistic activity encourages a pictorial expression of the inner experience that connects to the trauma in its own language, in a language of shapes, colors, and feelings. The artwork provides safe media for approaching the trauma since it is distant and outside the client's body. Sometimes children repeatedly recreate the trauma through art or play. This repeated processing of the traumatic experience can lead to relief, organization, and the finding of new strengths to deal with the disease. Sometimes, the body image is damaged as a result of illness or accident, and ways need to be found to deal with this. The goal of art therapy is to help the child cope with the change and the possible deformation of the body (Weinfeld-Yehoudayan, 2013).

Kaimal et al. (2019) emphasized the importance of educating patients and caregivers on the ways in which art therapy can help them cope with the challenges of treatment. Art therapy can help children prepare for a variety of medical procedures (surgeries, transplants, etc.). All the interviewees referred to different ways that have been developed over the years to prepare patients and sometimes also their parents for medical procedures. Painful medical procedures or devastating diagnoses are experienced as traumatic and art therapists can help the children and families process their experiences and foster greater resilience as they engage in treatment.

Another goal of art therapy is to enable the family to process their difficult experiences and help the child re-integrate with family and community in the best way possible (Weinfeld-Yehoudayan, 2013).

An art therapist who works at a rehabilitation hospital noted that the main goal is to shepherd these children back to a normative life as much as possible. In this hospital, art therapy takes place in a separate clinic which requires the children to leave their rooms to get there. The goal, in her view, is to restore the child's independence as much as possible, so she often works on acquiring abilities and practicing skills independently. In addition, she works on choices because dependence on parents often makes it difficult for these children to choose what they really want. When it comes to special education populations with lower levels of functioning, both in rehabilitation hospitals and in general hospitals, the transition to the hospital is often very confusing and the art therapist needs to help them cope emotionally.

The art therapists working in oncology wards emphasized the importance of accompanying children and families in dealing with the disease. A variety of issues and feelings can arise, so the goal in each session is to determine what is currently bothering the child and work with him/her in the "here and now". In addition, the course of the disease interjects other issues – some familial, some cultural – in relation to the parent–child relationship and in relation to the family's willingness to talk about the disease. In cases of children who are in terminal stages, the art therapist accompanies the child and the family, supports them, and allows them to say goodbye in a containing environment.

CHALLENGES

A number of art therapists addressed the difficulty of "courting" children. In fact, unlike in regular schools where the art therapist is assigned an orderly work plan, in the hospital every day begins anew with new and old patients and verifications of which patients need assistance and which patients will agree to engage in art therapy. Some art therapists actually described the act of "courtship" or "seduction" as they called it, in detail, which sometimes also includes starting an interaction via computer or tablet and hoping to continue the relationship by other means. One of the therapists said that the difficulty of courting children can be taxing. She takes little breaks to restore her energy and then returns with renewed strength. Sometimes art therapists cannot locate certain children who are in the midst of medical procedures, which results in lost time searching. This whole process demands a great deal of stamina.

All the art therapists made it clear that the treatment they provide in the hospital is secondary to medical care. They stressed that all children are in the hospital first and foremost to receive medical treatment and that any medical procedure takes priority over an art therapy session at any given time. One of the interviewees described an instance when a client had just shared something important and started crying when the doctor came in. This again points to the difficulties in creating and maintaining a safe therapeutic space.

One art therapist described the challenges involved in working with adolescents. She commented that adolescents, who are accustomed to a fairly large degree of independence, must revert to full close supervision by their parents in the hospital. The parents are suddenly much more exposed to the adolescent's behaviors, including the identity of phone callers and messages sent. They are also in a room where there are also other children and parents. The close quarters and supervision are difficult for these teenagers and can affect their willingness to cooperate.

An art therapist who works at a rehabilitation hospital described her feelings of despair when children do not seem to be progressing. Emotional changes can be very elusive and not always easy to characterize. This can lead to frustration. A number of art therapists talked about secondary trauma, which is now well-known in the literature, and the difficulties of dealing for years with the difficult stories and children suffering from pain. The trauma often enters into the personal lives of art therapists. Although most of them have worked for many years in hospital systems, some have described colleagues who could not stand the burden and sought employment elsewhere or retired.

Finally, art therapists working with children in terminal situations, such as in oncology wards, described the inconceivable difficulty of accompanying children to their deaths. This is compounded when parents do not authorize the therapist to talk to the child about impending death, even in situations where it is clear to the art therapist that the child is definitely aware of the situation. This also permeates their personal lives. One of the interviewees said that she hugs her children every time she comes home and thanks God for their health and that they are not in pain.

INTERVENTION TECHNIQUES AND DEDICATED WORKING MODELS

Working in an open space in hospitals (at the patient's bedside)

Weinfeld-Yehoudayan (2013) described ways to create an intimate work area in an open space in hospitals. The art therapist must offer his or her services such that these are not perceived as too intrusive or aggressive and obtain the patient's consent. Most of the time, children look forward to art therapy sessions, but sometimes due to physical pain or other reasons, they are not interested in having the session. In these cases, the patients should have the final say, and the therapist should cancel the session. The art therapist can offer an alternative time or date. In addition, the art therapist must be vigilant and adjust the duration of the session to the child's physical and medical condition. The duration of the session must be open to change, since there are various situations when the therapeutic session needs to be stopped in the middle or not started at all. Importantly, unlike classic art therapy, where clients do not need to be distracted, in the hospital, art therapy can help children temporarily "forget" physical pain, medication, and medical examinations.

In the open space of the hospital, the art therapy room is basically contained on a cart that is wheeled to the patient's bedside. The cart contains creative materials and games, which helps make it clear that the art therapist and the client can enter into a different space than the hospital ward that allows for experiences that once existed in the world outside the hospital. The figure of the art therapist and her/his cart can foster a relationship in which clients choose the materials or games they prefer and use them as they desire. Sometimes accessories related to a certain theme can be placed in the cart, such as broken objects that can lead to dealing with issues related to broken bones, loss, and trauma.

During a therapeutic session in an open space, restrained sublimation is sometimes required. In art therapy, this means creating on special trays with high sides, full aprons, and bedside tables to keep the patient and his/her environment clean, but also to allow expression through art materials. The entire creative process and therapeutic work are exposed to the staff and people near the patient's bed. Sometimes the child's condition requires intensive supervision by medical staff. This requires teamwork to help create separations and maintain the patient's privacy as much as possible. Weinfeld-Yehoudayan (2013) noted that although the creative product is not private, it is evident from the children's products that they go through a personal and private process that does not fall short of work created in a closed art therapy room.

Despite working in the open space, the art therapist needs to train his or her attention to be focused solely on the client. An explanation to the medical staff and family as to the importance of creating a therapeutic space can help. One of the art therapists said that despite the hospital's complex setting, during her work she discovered that there are many variations in a therapeutic relationship and that a meaningful and intimate relationship can be forged with a child even though the sessions are not regular and there are many interruptions. She found that through many short sessions, conversations and courtships, slowly and gradually, the minutes can accumulate and become a kind of container experience, and the therapeutic relationship can turn into something meaningful and deep.

Another art therapist addressed the importance of the fact that clients are often lying down when the art therapist approaches their bed. This position actually intensifies the clients' lack of control since they may find it difficult to end the session if something really does not suit them. In these situations, the therapist should be very careful about touching on traumatic experiences and should do so with measured inputs and exits and without forcing clients to dwell on these experiences. In this respect, the invitation to create in art materials can constitute a safe space for emotional inquiry to the extent appropriate for each client.

The need for great flexibility on the part of the art therapist

One of the art therapists stressed how diverse the setting can be within a hospital, which depends to a great extent on the child and family. She described how she sometimes does artwork with children even during medical procedures. For example, she mentioned a girl with burns who did artwork while having her bandage changed, which helped her be more relaxed and also increased her cooperation. In another instance, with another girl who was very anxious before surgery, they went on a walk together during which they also drew together, which helped her to relax.

Single session art therapy

One art therapist described a mode of intervention in the case of a single therapeutic session. Every morning she is given a list of the children in the ward, their ages, and the reason for hospitalization. The educator and the therapist decide together whom the art therapist should try to engage in therapeutic work. They go from bed to bed and talk to the children to identify where art therapy is needed, who can be in therapy in terms of pain levels, and how they can be recruited. They try to help in situations where patients are anxious before a medical procedure or when they express interest in art therapy. The work is always focused on the "here and now" and the art therapist tries to identify the nature of the need in the moment: are patients before or after a medical procedure, has something bothered them or disappointed them? (friends who did not call or someone who said that s/he was about to be released or was tired of staying in the ward...). The art intervention is tailored to the situation. For example, painting mandalas seems to have a calming effect, in particular since virtually any client can succeed. The more anxious the child is, the smaller the page should be and the more structured the work. Sometimes, the art therapist also introduces the client to cards that she has prepared specifically for focused work in the hospital. The cards have keywords such as "pain", "despair", "anxiety", "recovery", "support", or phrases to complete such as "no one can feel how much I....", "this hospitalization makes me..." and also pictures for example of doctors standing around a patient's bed or a nurse treating a child. The kit also includes pictures showing children engaging in normal activities such as at the beach, a group of friends chatting together, a dance, and others. These cards help the art therapist focus on the difficulties and start working. Once clients choose the cards that are right for them, they can be encouraged to create a work of art. With adolescents, the intervention often involves creating a collage that contains everything that currently bothers them. This single session actually helps to focus, give meaning, and clarify the patients' condition to them. It can sometimes calm and allow the expression of fears and anxieties.

Another art therapist indicated that in cases of a single session she sometimes incorporates CBT (cognitive behavioral therapy) interventions to help patients separate thoughts from emotions and look more deeply at what they are going through, depending on the patient's age and level of functioning. She sometimes uses an image of a balloon for the pain or for the anxiety. On the first day of hospitalization or medical procedure, the balloon is fully inflated, but later can shrink and can be better controlled. If it is appropriate for the patient to be involved in creative work, this process can be drawn.

Use of medical equipment in creative work

Many art therapists described how they search through medical equipment in storerooms and find all kinds of discarded equipment they can put to use in therapeutic work. One interviewee said that since the world of these children consists of a variety of medical procedures and medical equipment, to stimulate talk on this issue, the equipment itself must be part of what she presents to her clients. Clients can play with an anatomical doll or glue devices such as an old stethoscope or ace bandages or squirt water with modified syringes. Playing and creating artwork using medical equipment give children the opportunity to control devices that they usually have no control over. One art therapist described an anatomical doll she keeps permanently in her cart that has appealed to clients for years. It can be disassembled, washed, bandaged, etc. For example, she described a girl who underwent surgery and had the doll undergo the same operations. Another therapist said that she uses an anatomical doll when she prepares children for surgery.

Megides et al. (2009) described a working model with sick children in the hospital that was developed and built in collaboration with artist Hanoch Piven. They set up a workshop in the oncology ward of the hospital. The goal was to make this artist's way of working, which consists of making portraits out of unconventional objects, accessible to these patients (see link http://pivenworld.com/). In the workshop sessions, different types of materials reflecting worlds of content and texture such as wood, plastic, metal, fabric, and found materials from nature are set out on a central table. Medical equipment, such as syringes, infusion tubes, gloves, and masks, which are familiar objects to children and their families from the hospital world, are also included. The rationale is to allow sick children to work with the medical equipment from a position of choice and control as opposed to the helplessness, paralysis, intrusion, and pain that typically involve the use of these medical devices. The ability to play with the medical props and incorporate them into the artwork gives the children a chance to do what they want with these instruments and settle scores. These workshops highlight the potential of this technique for the expression and processing of difficult subjects, where the connection with the artist instills enthusiasm and a creative spirit.

Art therapy as support for children in painful procedures

Favara-Scacco et al. (2001) suggested the following procedure for children undergoing painful procedures: (1) *Clinical dialogue* – During each one-hour session, through specific questions, the therapist ascertains the client's behavioral style related to the immediate, unusual, and traumatic environment. Dialogue methodology differs as a function of client age. For children aged two to five years, for example, the therapist uses a puppet to promote a perception of the art therapist as a playful, "safe" person. (2) *Visual imagination* – Visual imagination is designed to support the child before the painful intervention. It activates an alternative thinking process. (3) *Medical play* – Medical play utilizes a cloth doll and medical instruments to allow age-appropriate explanations about the procedure. The child's need to reject explanations perceived as overwhelming is respected. (4) *Structured drawing* – Structured drawing is utilized with children who exhibit a great need for control. A sheet of paper printed with the outline of a drawing is given to the client to color. Structured drawing provides an organized external reality (the drawing) and can be helpful in reducing anxiety and tension. (5) *Redundant reading* – Redundant reading is specific to preschoolers. Reading a story over and over stimulates a sense of control comparable to that of a structured drawing. (6) *Free drawing* – Free drawing is used for children who need to liberate their inner imaginations. It helps the child externalize and get rid of internal confusion by "casting" it on a sheet of white paper. (7) *Dramatization* – Dramatization is used for children who need to "act out" their anxiety, release, and lessen it through movement.

Art therapy for children in oncology wards

Over the years, greater numbers of oncology wards in Israel have begun to offer art therapy. The art therapists who work in these wards emphasized that the intervention is always specific to family and culture. Art therapists from both Jewish and Arab cultures in Israel made it clear that it is the right of every family to decide what to tell a child at different stages of the disease, and that they accompany the process in the way the family chooses. There are families who agree to talk freely about the disease and its meaning, while other families choose not to tell the child or at times the family circle to save face and preserve family status. The art therapists stated that they attempted to persuade these families to be open about the disease in the belief that it was better for the child's mental health and the mental health of other family members, but that the final decision was up to them. In oncology wards, treatment can last several months. The art therapy sessions are given in the suitable place for each child, either at the bedside or in the art therapy room. The interviewees talked about the difficulty of creating a sense of safe space and continuity in treatment, because the therapeutic session is often interrupted or disrupted by external needs, such as staff members taking the patient for a variety of medical procedures, or internal factors such as pain or weakness, which prevent the child from engaging in the sessions. During the therapeutic session, children are invited to work with art materials. If they are in bed, they are asked what materials they want, and the art therapist brings them in the cart. The artwork helps children express the range of complex emotions surrounding the disease including the fear of death that is sometimes difficult to talk about. The expression itself helps to alleviate loneliness while reinforcing the feeling that there is room for these feelings as well. When children need to be in isolation in the hospital, art therapists try to produce a sterile kit they can take with them. When they have to go through medical procedures such as radiation, transplants, and others, the art therapists often prepare a diary they can keep during this period where they can draw and write about their experiences and how they are doing.

One art therapist described the joint development by a team of art therapists in an oncology ward of a protocol to prepare young children for radiation therapy. Radiation therapy is administered in the radiation unit and requires the young child to lie still. To avoid daily anesthesia, the protocol consisted of several sessions in which the young child and his/her parents use play and guided imagery to practice lying motion-less for several minutes (the sculpture game) and develop the ability to stay by themselves in the accelerator without their parents (the joint thought game). This preparation was carried out in collaboration with parents and staff of the radiation unit. The staff also prepared illustrated instruction booklets for children and parents.

Art therapy in a rehabilitation hospital

In rehabilitation hospitals, the situation is somewhat different since the patients by definition stay several months. Art therapy is usually held twice a week and aims at promoting independence and helping the patients return as much as possible to their previous lives under new conditions. In order to meet these goals, when patients come to the art therapy room, they are presented with the art materials and are invited to work in the way that suits them best. Sometimes, they are invited to create with the art therapist. One art therapist noted that it is often difficult for these children to create with art materials. In her opinion, art can add extra tension, perhaps because of the difficulty of motor performance as compared to their proficiency before the injury, or because of the difficulty playing and expressing themselves as a result of the trauma. She thus often works with them in very primary ways such as color mixing, color games without products, scribbles, and the like. On the other hand, when she feels that these children are capable of creating and expanding their repertoire, she will try to push them to do so, to increase their skills and come closer to independent activities. The products all remain in the art therapy room so that there is a feeling of something preserved and protected, which is not always the case in the hospital at large.

Open studio

One of the art therapists described group artwork within the wards using an open studio setting that allows children to come and create. Sometimes, the work can be structured, such as working on masks or personal portraits or on individual or group mandalas. At other times, tables can be laid out with different topics or different materials. Kaimal et al. (2019) noted that open art studios in outpatient infusion centers, where most young cancer and blood disorder patients receive much of their care, can promote an atmosphere of safety and inclusion, maximize patients' choices, and provide nonverbal avenues to communicate feelings and needs to the medical team. In this case, the art therapists hold open studios during clinic hours and invite all the patients and caregivers to participate, thus normalizing the treatment experience and diminishing the isolation of cancer treatment.

THE MEANING OF ART

A number of art therapists argued that art for sick children is the healthy component that connects them to their places of strength. Art provides an authentic opportunity to create, play, and express themselves. Art is also familiar and is something they remember from kindergarten or school when they were healthy as part of their daily routine. Art making enables a connection to internal sources of creation, and in this case to the healthy forces of life and healing. These components often help patients cope with the disease. In addition, art helps to express emotions that are difficult to express in words such as anger, frustration, fear, and disappointment.

Most art therapists mentioned the calming element of art for sick children. Sometimes calming is required before or even during medical procedures and incorporating art making can moderate the degree of trauma experienced by the child undergoing treatment. Art is one of the only ways that leaves a tangible product behind, a fingerprint in the world. The clients' work is a visual and external documentation of the self, which is especially significant in life-threatening circumstances. In cases of terminal illness, the artistic product remains as lasting evidence of the child's existence.

COLLABORATIVE INTERVENTIONS INVOLVING PARENTS AND STAFF MEMBERS

Working with parents

The relationship with parents in hospitals is crucial because they decide what information will be passed on to the child and what content they agree to discuss. One of the art therapists stated honestly that she starts from the premise that if her children were hospitalized, she would never let a stranger approach them. Therefore, in her view, her initial relationship must be with the parents. Sometimes parents allow therapeutic sessions with the child to take place in their absence, but other times insist on their presence. In some cases, the art therapist suggests joint work with the art materials to reassure both the child and the family. In addition, hospitalization often challenges the parent–child relationship due to the intensity of their time together and parental control over the child's life, so that many art therapists find themselves in the position of mediator between parents and children.

In the oncology ward, where relationships with patients are longer, contact with the parents is much more important. The parents themselves sometimes turn to the art therapist when they need a moment to share, unload, cry, or consult. In some situations, parents also join sessions with their children. For example, one art therapist described an adolescent client whose cancer had returned, which caused great emotional distress. In one of the art therapy sessions, she asked the mother to come in with her. During the therapy session, she dealt with the question of whether she was allowed to be afraid and cry. When the therapist replied that of course it was allowed, the client began to cry and said how afraid and apprehensive she was about the surgery she was about to undergo. Her mother listened to all this dialogue, took a deep breath, and told her that she believed that everything was in the hands of God, who had already taken her out of this disease once. She began reading verses from the Koran that seemed to her might reassure her child as well as herself. The client listened patiently, looked at her mother, and suddenly calmed down. The art therapist thus helped the client and her mother, this time without art materials, to create another bond in a safe place, that gave the daughter some peace.

When dealing with a life-threatening illness, alongside feelings of chaos, fear, anger, damage to image and self-worth, as well as loss of control, children experience immense loneliness. Loneliness is related to being sick in front of others, the healthy ones, and the difficulty of sharing thoughts that everyone has but will not utter: the fear of death. Children are preoccupied with death even if they eventually recover from the disease. Death is shrouded in taboo, all the more so when it comes to the death of children. Parents and children share a mutual desire to protect one other. This leaves everyone alone with fears and thoughts as to what might happen. The language of art makes it possible to symbolically express and process threatening feelings that are frightening to talk about directly and consciously. The metaphorical work allows for a dimension of externalization which reduces the threats of reality and allows for painful content to be voiced. For example, an eight-year-old client created a doll in art therapy that kept falling apart. Her body was unstable, the hair she was pasting on constantly fell out, and her hands fell off. Throughout the session, she got upset and expressed frustration and anger that nothing was working for her, nothing was going as she had planned, and everything was falling apart and was damaged. Finally, she built a box that looked like a coffin. She padded the box from the inside, laid the doll in it, and said: "Here she can't fall apart, because no one will touch her anymore, and she can rest".

One of the art therapists described support groups for siblings in the oncology ward that are led by the art therapist and another staff member. In these groups, siblings are given a place to express what they are going through, in a supportive framework in which everyone feels similarly. The contents that come up in these groups involve feelings of loneliness, anxiety, sadness, anger, jealousy and guilt, and very great concern. At times, the sick child invites the siblings to attend an art therapy session. These encounters are very meaningful and allow the siblings to process the relationship between them, and sometimes even constitute a protected space for separation processes.

In rehabilitation hospitals, the art therapist meets once every two weeks with the parents without the child. This art therapist noted that since all the parents are going through very difficult events with their children, the parental training concentrates on post-trauma. She often uses art-based interventions when working with parents. For example, she asks them to draw an image that represents the child to them and then represent their relationship. Observing the work opens up different facets of their perception of both the child and their relationship. Sometimes, especially in cases where the parent–child relationship is strained or the parent finds it hard to cope with the child's condition, she asks the parent and child to take part in parent–child art psychotherapy. She noted that especially in cases of brain injury, the adjustment can be very confusing for the parent since the child looks the same, but his/her functioning is very different than before the injury.

The relationship between the medical and the educational–therapeutic staff varies considerably from ward to ward. Over time, there has been a greater appreciation of the role of arts therapy in wards in hospitals in the State of Israel. Nevertheless, considerable differences remain. The art therapists interviewed here felt that the closest teamwork occurred in oncology wards, where meetings of the entire staff are organized regularly to discuss the ongoing care of each patient, both medical and educational–therapeutic.

At times, there can also be differences in orientations between the therapeutic staff and the educational staff mainly due to a lack of a clear definition of roles. Special education teachers often do not actually teach academic material in hospitals and tend to drift into the role of arts therapists. This can blur the distinction between a professional who has degrees in arts therapy and another who has simply acquired techniques from field experience.

The therapeutic staff also provides emotional support to the educational and medical staff. Based on a concept presented by Megides et al. (2009), workshops can also be designed for staff members. Staff members can rest and vent emotions in these art workshops and by making portraits using objects.

CLINICAL ILLUSTRATION

Three months have elapsed since 11-year-old Daniel was diagnosed with cancer. During these three months, his life has turned upside down and he now spends increasingly more days a month in the hospital. He has a hard time remembering his previous life because the experiences are so intense and shaky. Some days he felt like he is on a wild roller coaster ride he has no control over. He tries very hard to keep in touch with classmates but feels day by day how different his life had become from theirs. They talk to him about school, about classes, about friends while he is busy with a variety of tests and medical efforts to treat his illness.

Daniel's family has also undergone a significant shake-up. His parents do shifts at his bedside, with one parent always with him while the other parent tries to handle life at home, where two other younger sisters are waiting for them. His parents have told Daniel he is ill but try very hard to keep his hopes up. Not a word has been said about pains and difficulties. Dad tries to entertain him and make him laugh with a variety of funny stories and videos. Mom plays board games with him and sings songs to him when he feels less good.

Daniel was offered art therapy as soon as he entered the hospital, but it took two to three weeks before he agreed to start. The art therapist would typically come to his bedside with a cart full of varied art materials. Daniel had already forgotten when he had last painted and he felt it was no longer appropriate for his age, but he was intrigued by a huge basket of strange objects that were at the bottom of the cart. He and Dad took out the objects and hung or draped them on themselves in a funny way each time creating a more interesting and stranger image. The art therapist looked at them and smiled. She suggested that they take a sheet of cardboard and stick the objects on it to make a portrait. While explaining the task to them, Nili, a nurse in the hospital, peeked into the room to check that everything was okay, and that Daniel's infusion was still dripping correctly. Nili had funny glasses and a weird scarf around her neck. When she left, Dad started giggling as did Daniel. Almost without words, the two began to make her portrait from the objects in the basket. Although Daniel was weak and at times in pain, the joint art activity helped distract him. When they finished, they showed the work to other patients in the ward and asked them to say who they thought the picture was about.

The art therapy sessions continued throughout the following weeks, depending on Daniel's condition. Sometimes he was happy to see the art therapist but other times he was too weak. When the sessions took place, Daniel made other portraits of everyone around him: family members, other patients, and especially the staff. Everyone was waiting for Daniel's artwork, which made them happy and cheerful; one by one he hung them over his bed. However, as the days went by, the art therapist felt that she had only reached the tip of the iceberg. The art made Daniel very happy and helped distract him from his weakness and pain, and also raised his self-confidence when all those around him admired his works. However, the art therapist had a feeling that so far only positive feelings of joy and laughter and perhaps distraction had been accessed. The more difficult feelings had not yet been expressed and processed in any way. She asked Daniel's parents to meet her without Daniel.

In a session with the parents, the art therapist saw two tired, suffering people, who appeared to be very different from their behavior at

Daniel's bedside. Although Daniel's condition was not yet clear, the prognosis was difficult and required mental strength from them. In the session, they dared talk about their pain and at one point Daniel's mother burst into tears. The art therapist listened, tried to help as much as she could, and finally also expressed her opinion that Daniel also needed to find a way to express his difficult feelings. She asked to see Daniel in the art therapy room without his parents present.

The following week Daniel felt well enough one day to go with the art therapist to her room. He discovered a vast amount of art materials, games, and also a basket of medical equipment that caught his attention. The art therapist showed him how to combine medical equipment with art materials. They found a syringe, put paint in it and Daniel made several attempts to control the amount of paint coming out of the syringe and draw a picture with it. Slowly and carefully, he drew the sky and then added the sun. He changed colors attentively and tried to direct the color to the right places. At the bottom of the paper, he added soil and a puddle of water with some grass around it. The color was slightly diffused, but the resulting images could certainly be identified. The last task was drawing a fish to swim in the pond. Daniel was very focused and slowly created the shape of the fish. He paused for a moment and then added a small eye to it. He smiled and said he was pleased. After finishing, the art therapist and Daniel looked at the painting. It was a simple drawing but the fish in the pond stood out in its solitude. The art therapist was debating whether to say anything. As they observed the painting, wind from the window wafted over the drying painting and the drop of the eye moved slightly and trickled down. The fish seemed to be crying. Daniel watched what was happening and tears flowed down his cheeks. It was clear that he, too, saw the loneliness of the fish. The art therapist put a hand on his shoulder and cautiously began to talk to him about the fish's feelings and in subsequent sessions, his own feelings.

SUMMARY

Art therapy with students in the hospital for a variety of medical conditions is unique and different from anything discussed so far. The main goals include first and foremost an attempt to help these clients regain control in situations where they are experiencing uncontrollable events such as invasive testing and procedures. Art can help encourage distraction and produce a sense of control at least in this space. In addition, many patients experience trauma and losses before and during hospitalization, which can begin to be expressed and processed through art. Art therapists can also help prepare for a variety of medical procedures, sometimes with art materials. It is important to remember that the family is also present and often the treatment will also include helping the whole family deal with the illness and the difficulties that accompany it. In rehabilitation hospitals, efforts are made to encourage the client to regain independence and return to as many previous functions as possible. In oncology wards, art therapists accompany the client and family in the complex coping with the disease, and sometimes in the separation processes leading to death.

A number of major challenges facing art therapists in hospitals were discussed. The therapists talked about the processes of "courtship" and "seduction" in trying to recruit patients for art therapy sessions. These processes require considerable investment in energy and sometimes cause burnout. In addition, they are aware that the treatment they give will always be a second priority with respect to medical treatment, which leads to interruptions even in the middle of sessions. Sometimes, especially in adolescents, there is a great deal of resistance due to the symbiotic conditions that occur as a result of the disease and that can cause considerable anger. In rehabilitation hospitals, the processes are very slow, and improvement is measured on a micro-scale. Above all, most art therapists referred to the secondary trauma that affects their lives as a result of exposure to these difficult situations, which sometimes end by accompanying clients to their death.

Working in hospitals challenges the traditional setting of art therapy. Sometimes, sessions are held in open spaces by the patient's bedside while trying to maintain an experience of intimacy as much as possible. This unique setting requires major adjustments in terms of ways to create privacy, such as bringing the art materials to the bedside and maintaining cleanliness within the hygienic setting of a hospital. The interviewees stressed that they are called on to show flexibility, and they find themselves altering or violating the therapeutic setting in almost every possible way and even enabling clients to do artwork during medical procedures. When art therapy only involves a single session, the art therapists sometimes use cards or other techniques that they have developed over the years to focus the therapeutic encounter. They all said that they work in the "here and now" because the reality in the hospital can change from day to day and from hour to hour. They aim to support clients by preparing them for medical procedures and when they are in pain. Sometimes they do so by using medical and hospital equipment and devices to increase the client's sense of control. Sometimes, they run an open studio, where patients, their parents, and also staff members can take part and express their feelings through art. In oncology wards, they tailor the treatment to each family and accompany each client and family in the way that best corresponds to their battle with the disease, and sometimes also assists in separation processes when medical treatment has not been successful. In rehabilitation hospitals, they help clients regain habits and functions to recover some degree of independence.

REFERENCES

Aguilar, B. A. (2017). The efficacy of art therapy in pediatric oncology patients: An integrative literature review. *Journal of Pediatric Nursing, 36*, 173–178.

Clapp, L. A., Taylor, E. P., Di Folco, S., & Mackinnon, V. L. (2019). Effectiveness of art therapy with pediatric populations affected by medical health conditions: A systematic review. *Arts & Health, 11*(3), 183–201.

Councill, T. D., & Ramsey, K. (2019). Art therapy as a psychosocial support in a Child's palliative care. *Art Therapy, 36*(1), 40–45.

Favara-Scacco, C., Smirne, G., Schilirò, G., & Di Cataldo, A. (2001). Art therapy as support for children with leukemia during painful procedures. *Medical and Pediatric Oncology: The Official Journal of SIOP—International Society of Pediatric Oncology (Societé Internationale d'Oncologie Pédiatrique, 36*(4), 474–480.

Kaimal, G., Councill, T., Ramsey, K., Cottone, C., & Snyder, K. (2019). A conceptual framework for approaches to art therapy research in paediatric hematology/oncology settings. *Canadian Art Therapy Association Journal, 32*(2), 95–103.

Malchiodi, C. A. (2013). *Art therapy and health care.* Guilford Press.

Megides, O., Shalev, J., Trismann, S., Koren, Y., & Piven, H. (2009). Drawing with readymade objects: A model for therapeutic workshops integrating art and group therapy. *Bein-Hamilim,* 1, 1–9. (In Hebrew).

Metzl, E., Morrell, M., & Field, A. (2016). A pilot outcome study of art therapy and music therapy with hospitalized children (Étude pilote des résultats de l'art-thérapie et de la musicothérapie auprès d'enfants hospitalisés). *Canadian Art Therapy Association Journal, 29*(1), 3–11.

Raybin, J. L., & Krajicek, M. (2020). Creative arts therapy in the context of children with cancer: A concept analysis. *Journal of Pediatric Oncology Nursing, 37*(2), 82–90.

Reed, K., Kennedy, H., & Wamboldt, M. Z. (2015). Art for life: A community arts mentorship program for chronically ill children. *Arts & Health, 7*(1), 14–26.

Stafstrom, C. E., Havlena, J., & Krezinski, A. J. (2012). Art therapy focus groups for children and adolescents with epilepsy. *Epilepsy & Behavior, 24*(2), 227–233.

Stinley, N. E., Norris, D. O., & Hinds, P. S. (2015). Creating mandalas for the management of acute pain symptoms in pediatric patients. *Art Therapy*, 32(2), 46–53.

Weinfeld-Yehoudayan, A. (2013). Unique characteristics of therapeutic work in an open space: Arts therapies in a hospital for children in the hemodialysis unit. *Academic Journal of Creative Arts Therapies*, 3(1), 273–285. (In Hebrew).

Wigham, S., Watts, P., Zubala, A., Jandial, S., Bourne, J., & Hackett, S. (2020). Using arts-based therapies to improve mental health for children and young people with physical health long-term conditions: A systematic review of effectiveness. *Frontiers in Psychology*, 11, 1771.

BRIEF BIOGRAPHIES OF THE ART THERAPISTS WHO CONTRIBUTED TO THIS CHAPTER

Micaela Amati, art therapist (M.A.) and supervisor, has worked for 22 years as an art therapist, including 20 years in special education settings for hospitalized students in a rehabilitation hospital.

Nibal Khoury, art therapist (M.A.), has worked for four years as an art therapist, including two years in special education settings for hospitalized students in the Schneider Children's Medical Center.

Idit Kravitz, art therapist (M.A.) and supervisor, has worked for 23 years as an art therapist, including 20 years in special education settings for hospitalized students.

Zakiah Massarwa, art therapist (M.A.) and supervisor, lecturer at the Bar-Ilan University, has worked for 23 years as an art therapist, including 14 years in special education settings for hospitalized students.

Orna Megides, art therapist (Psy.D.) and supervisor, lecturer at the School of Creative Arts Therapies at the University of Haifa, has worked for 23 years as an art therapist, including 7 years as an art therapist in the haemato-oncology ward of the Schneider Children's Medical Center.

Miriam Rish, art therapist and supervisor, has worked for 24 years as an art therapist, including 13 years in special education settings for hospitalized students.

Asnat Weinfeld-Yehoudayan, art therapist (M.A.), currently a Ph.D. student, and supervisor, has worked for 17 years as an art therapist in special education settings for hospitalized students at Shaare Zedek Medical Center.

Eight

INTRODUCTION

Child and adolescent art therapy mental health services settings can enable these clients to cope with their overwhelming experiences by identifying feelings non-verbally. Art therapy can help children and teens express an experience, fragmented or otherwise, beyond their declarative memories. One of the key underlying hypotheses of many therapeutic approaches, including art therapy, is that individuals' inability to adequately verbalize their traumatic experiences and associated emotions cause psychological problems to persist; thus, finding the words is a key step in therapy (Nielsen et al., 2019).

Lyshak-Stelzer et al. (2007) pointed out that for many years, art therapists have observed that drawing and painting can contribute to the assessment and treatment of traumatic disorders in children and adolescents. Because verbal recollection of the trauma is often difficult or beyond a child's capacity, approaches that do not rely heavily on verbal access to trauma material, such as art therapy, have exceptional value. Specifically, these authors reported a significant treatment-by-condition interaction where adolescents in the trauma-focused expressive art therapy protocol condition experienced a greater drop in post-traumatic stress disorder (PTSD) symptoms severity than adolescents in the treatment-as-usual condition. More recently, Ugurlu et al. (2016) assessed the effect of an art therapy intervention on post-traumatic stress, depression, and anxiety symptoms in Syrian refugee children ($N = 64$) and found that art therapy could help lessen these symptoms.

In a systematic meta-analysis, Braito et al. (2021) reviewed the evidence on art therapy and art psychotherapy in children receiving mental health services. The 17 articles are classified into two groups: 10 publications dealing with the treatment of children with a psychiatric

DOI: 10.4324/9781003156918-8

diagnosis, and seven publications on the treatment of children with psychiatric symptoms but no formal diagnosis. These studies vary in terms of the type of art therapy/psychotherapy delivered, the underlying conditions, and the outcome measures. Many are case studies/case series, or small quasi-experimental studies; there are few randomized control trials and no replication studies. Nevertheless, there is some evidence that art therapy or art psychotherapy can benefit children who have experienced trauma or who manifest PTSD symptoms.

Tyson and Baffour (2004) reported that many adolescents in an acute-care psychiatric setting tend to use arts-based methods to cope with the trauma in their daily lives. Some play musical instruments or listen to music, while others engage in writing and artwork (e.g., sculpting, drawing, painting, etc.). One of the most interesting aspects of these findings is that the arts-based methods described by the clients in this study were self-identified, and hence were interpreted as "youth strengths".

This chapter overviews the entire range of care of students with mental disorders in the education system and covers schools in psychiatric wards in hospitals and special schools for students diagnosed by a psychiatrist. At adulthood, these students tend to be classified as schizophrenic, or coping with personality disorders, depression, anxiety, and/or post-trauma. Some of these students are hospitalized in a psychiatric ward after attempting suicide. In these hospitals, clients are often categorized in terms of the level of functioning. Clients who pose a danger to themselves or to others are hospitalized in closed wards. Some are considered capable of attending a special school in the ward whereas others remain under full supervision and are treated by the art therapist individually in their room. Clients who do not pose a danger to themselves or others are sometimes hospitalized in open wards or in a psychiatric day hospital. Special schools for students with mental disorders in the community accept students with a psychiatric diagnosis who cannot be integrated into a regular school, and sometimes go in and out of hospitals.

One of the art therapists working at a special school for students with mental disorders in the community said she identifies two major groups of students. The first is composed of extroverted students, who often present with attention-deficit hyperactivity disorder (ADD/ADHD) or oppositional defiant disorder (ODD) with very severe regulation problems. These students always take up a lot of space in the school, react to every event, and are often involved in social incidents. The second group is introverted students, who are often diagnosed with anxiety or depression. These students often avoid others, do not leave the classroom, and become isolated.

In addition, a population of students copes with eating disorders. In the State of Israel, if hospitalization is required, these students are referred to designated wards that specialize in eating disorders. A few years ago, together with Prof. Sharon Snir from Tel Hai College and with the professional support of Pazit Carmon, an art therapist and supervisor, we supervised a thesis by a student, Rotem Ben-Gal Hazan (who has since become an art therapist in her own right) on the topic of art therapy with clients with eating disorders. The data gathered in this study was based on interviews with art therapists working with these clients as well as case descriptions from publications in the field (Acharya et al., 1995; Beck, 2007; Edwards, 2008; Harnden, 1995; Jeong & Kim, 2006; Malchiodi, 1999; Matto, 1997; Naitove, 1986; Schaverien, 1994; Wolf et al., 1986). Since this study was only published in Hebrew (in the *Academic Journal of Creative Arts Therapies* belonging to the Emili Sagol Research Center at the School of Creative Arts Therapies at the University of Haifa) (Ben-Gal Hazan et al., 2019), I summarize some of the findings in this chapter, with the approval of the Journal.

THE THERAPEUTIC GOALS OF ART THERAPY

The art therapists interviewed for this chapter all concurred that the main goal of working with these clients is to improve their quality of life, maximize their ability to integrate into society in the best way possible in the future, and in many cases also attempt to help them choose life over death. One interviewee made it clear that the goal is first and foremost authentic expression via art making and the integration of the forces of creation and the client's difficulties, problems, distortions, and traumas. In hospitals, however, due to the need to quickly discharge children and adolescents, the goal is often reduced to stabilizing the situation before returning home. The message is nevertheless conveyed that it is okay to be hospitalized for a certain amount of time and that the range of experiences these clients have undergone and the difficulties they have experienced are above and beyond what children or adolescents can go through unsupported on their own. In day hospitalizations in hospitals or special schools in the community, the goal can be expanded to returning to the best level of functioning possible.

One art therapist who works in a closed ward felt that art therapy in this type of ward gives adolescents a space where they can create and be heard, and express their inner worlds, fantasies, and feelings, which take shape and color through the artistic process. Art is an "island of sanity" in the midst of chaos and madness, where hardships and difficulties arise but also the discovery of strengths. Behind the manifestations of the trauma and illness, there are life stories, hopes, and aspirations, as well as unconscious areas that have not been expressed. Working with children and adolescents with mental disorders can fluctuate between their intense urges to express themselves and the need for defense at all costs. In the artistic process, defensive and adaptive behaviors occur simultaneously. Sometimes their art departs from conventions. In their works, there are constant deviations from the norms and criteria of color organization and materiality. The artworks can be very powerful, conveying deep and moving emotions. The style is completely subjective at times, suggesting that breaking the rules is sometimes the message itself.

The interviewees all referred to the therapeutic alliance they formed with their clients, sometimes during lengthy treatment, that helps the clients feel that they are indeed meaningful to someone else. Creating a therapeutic alliance is a goal in itself that is constantly worked on throughout all stages of therapy. For art therapists, the goal is to create a relationship that will allow for meaningful connections, regression to dependence, and the processing of past traumas in the most beneficial ways. However, many clients fail to form this kind of relationship. In schools for students with mental disorders in the community, attempts are made to allow clients to continue with the same art therapist over the entire course of their education to enable a continuous and stable relationship to form. The therapeutic alliance can nevertheless be challenged at times when clients see that other students have also made significant contact with their therapist.

One of the art therapists working at a special school in the community described the goals in the form of stages. In the first stage when a new student arrives, the main goal is adaptation as well as acceptance. The student needs to both adapt to the new framework and also accept the fact that s/he corresponds to the population of this school. Most sessions in the first year or two deal with the meaning of the diagnosis, the accompanying stigma, and the need to be in a specialized setting. Since the school integrates students with very different psychiatric diagnoses, new students also try to position themselves with respect to their similarities and differences with others. In the next stage, the goal involves accepting the psychiatric diagnosis. Students must grapple with issues related to the ways in which the diagnosis defines them and how to live with their disability. Questions also arise in relation to medication. Some want to know the root cause (a traumatic event, heredity, and others). They slowly begin to engage with life itself and their peer group. Toward the end of treatment, the next goal is preparing for post-school life. Some choose national service, further education, or the job market. Some move to a hostel. Other issues also affect these stages such as spates of hospitalizations.

Another goal relates to creating and strengthening a sense of belonging and togetherness in group work. Some of these students become extremely lonely when they feel no hope can come from their environment. Working in a group setting allows for an experience of togetherness and contact through the artistic process. Even for severe cases of students who are unable to give meaning to their work, engaging in art in the presence of others allows for an experience of belonging and trust.

Clients with eating disorders (Ben-Gal Hazan et al., 2019)

Most art therapists and several of the articles reviewed in this study noted the need for clients to understand that an eating disorder does not always disappear completely and that clients need to learn to live alongside the eating disorder, understand the symptoms, and what they are telling them. The goal of art therapy is to allow clients to minimize their preoccupation with the body and expand their world so that the eating disorder takes up less space in their lives. This goal addresses not only the need to learn to live with the symptoms themselves, but also the ways art therapy can help clients in other areas of life affected by the eating disorder to improve their quality of life. In art therapy, clients are invited to explore the difficulties and problems they face and seek out effective solutions where the clients can achieve the best of themselves.

Most of the interviewees and half of the articles reviewed in the study showed that mental inflexibility and rigidity characterize clients coping with anorexia. In this case, the goal of art therapy is to achieve more flexibility with respect to perfectionism, object permanence, and the need for control and restrictions. Expansion through the use of art materials can contribute to relaxing these restrictions and these clients' dichotomous view of the world. Art making can provide room for experiences, feelings, and emotions that have been blurred by anorexia. Clients are encouraged to enter a creative space to let go of rigid and incessant speech and allow for spontaneity and passion.

Another key goal emerging from most interviews and about half of the articles is the need to teach these clients how to cope and express their eating disorders and symptoms non-somatically. The sessions are structured to provide moments of respite that involve transferring the preoccupation with food to art and art materials. This dialogue is developed during the treatment to enable the client to apply it to situations outside the art therapy room. The treatment allows clients to find strengths within themselves and begin to face difficulties that have not yet found expression in words. The internal dialogue becomes a visual dialogue that can be talked about and yields insights that enable effective coping.

Most of the articles reviewed in this study emphasized the importance of expressing emotions, given these clients' difficulties expressing themselves emotionally. The goal of therapy is to use art as a way to explore feelings and emotions and deal with difficulties. The emotions revealed through art are often very difficult to disclose to oneself or to others. Art therapy can allow some of the emotional expression to remain on the page without a need to talk about it.

CHALLENGES

The art therapists described the difficult cases they work with, including children or adolescents who have been sexually abused or the victims of incest. These are compelling and frightening cases that can affect their personal lives. They described their need to relax, including holding supervision, or pastimes that calm them down. Some described violence on the ward and the fear of imminent outbursts, which makes it difficult to form a therapeutic alliance. One of the art therapists working in a psychiatric ward with children with Autism Spectrum

Disorder (ASD) said that she positions a table between her and the client such that she is near the door in case of need. In other situations, clients are unable to stay in the art therapy room because the intimate relationship threatens them and simply leave after a few minutes.

One of the art therapists who works in a closed ward stated that the psychotic processes make it difficult to create a relationship between the art therapist and the client in which trust can develop and emotions can be dealt with. Sometimes a form of courtship is required to overcome resistance, until a client is ready to go to the art therapy room. Other interviewees described their difficulties working with parents, who also often come from difficult backgrounds and can create splits and projections in the staff. In other cases, working with parents is frustrating when they do not cooperate or do not advance in the therapeutic process.

Some art therapists working in hospitals described their attempts to allow a wide variety of instruments, including those that cut in the art therapy room, and how difficult it is to monitor and be responsible for safety. Scissors, sharpeners, and other tools need to be marked and counted after each session. One of the art therapists reported that some clients want to use their own blood in their artwork, which she prohibits because she believes that within hospitalization, it is not something that can be allowed.

Clients with eating disorders (Ben-Gal Hazan et al., 2019)

Most art therapists and about half of the articles reviewed in the study talked about problems at the beginning of treatment making contact, which usually communicated the difficulty of wanting change and dealing with the eating disorder. This makes building a therapeutic alliance highly important, which can be facilitated at times through art making. In other cases, the resistance is to the art making. Mistrust and fears in therapy correspond to the feeling that the world is not a safe place. Some art therapists indicated that if the therapeutic alliance is not formed quickly, clients may drop out. Even after initial contact has been made, clients may abandon treatment to avoid feeling exposed or having to open up.

Most art therapists and a few of the articles reviewed in the study characterized clients, especially those coping with anorexia, as manifesting stiffness, reduction, and perfectionism, whose entire world has been reduced to weight and calorie counting. Through their preoccupation and reduction of food intake, they can have a sense of control over the body and at times over others. The art therapists felt that the anorexic client's world was first reduced physically but that this can also be seen in unregulated emotional and mental expressions that arise during treatment. Despite its contribution to relaxing certain rigid patterns, some interviewees noted that these clients find art making difficult as a result of their perfectionism and their experience of "all or nothing".

INTERVENTION TECHNIQUES AND DEDICATED WORKING MODELS

Dynamic individual art therapy

All the art therapists interviewed reported that they took an open and dynamic work approach with their clients. They described how they invite clients to work freely with the art materials. Occasionally, they will put out a particular material or suggest a particular technique to help expand the client's repertoire. One of the art therapists said that in her view, "children who break down do not need art materials that break down". Instead, in the ward where she works, she insists that the art materials she provides to clients are of high quality and in good condition. A number of art therapists stated that they tend to use more solid materials (such as pencils, oil pastels, and markers) and put more regressive and liquid materials in the closet. Other art therapists noted that even when the art materials are all displayed to the clients, they usually prefer to start working with more solid materials and only later dare try more regressive art materials, sometimes after interventions from the art therapist designed to expand their use of art materials.

One of the art therapists who works in a psychiatric day ward said that she only works with a few art materials but of very high quality, because she believes that art therapy should give these clients the possibility of really working in art. The creative process is central in her art therapy room and she tries to encourage art making through high-quality materials. She tries not to provide art therapy to adolescents who are artists, to avoid interfering with their spontaneous art making, and transfers them to another therapist who works in different modalities. However, the clients who do come to her slowly learn the language of art. She hangs sheets of different sizes and shapes on the easels and places a palette of gouache paints (basic colors, black, white, and brown), three different size brushes, a jar of water, and a towel. High-quality art materials are placed on the table such as pastel sticks, chalks, markers, watercolors, natural charcoal, pencils, newspapers, glue, and clay. She does not provide any craft materials at all, since she believes that working with them does not correspond to an in-depth exploration of the mind. During the first sessions, she applies Edith Kramer's intake approach. She asks the client to create three artworks. The first is made with clay or gouache. The second involves working with the art material that was not chosen for the first work. The third consists of work on a sheet of A4 paper with a pencil. She tells clients that everything they do is okay and that there is no right or wrong. If clients refuse, she invites them to engage in joint drawing games. In any case, she also suggests joint artworks to clients in the intake stage. She also suggests all kinds of games with the art materials (e.g., clients make a shape and she paints inside it, after which they reverse roles, finger games with gouache in order to encourage clients to work with the material, etc.). During the artwork, she observes whether the client's work is developing in the sense of learning to mix colors, make different patterns, etc. This observation is also informative as to the way the client makes contact with her. The goal is to eventually achieve independent artistic creation with a variety of art materials.

One art therapist described in depth how clients' attitudes toward art materials can tell so much about them. Some clients need to be almost seduced by a variety of art materials to get them to engage in artwork. Other clients use excessive amounts of art materials, almost swallowing them, and never feel satiated. The feeling, she said, was that in a moment they would swallow the room, and devour her as well, and it still would not be enough.

A number of art therapists commented that some pieces of equipment are always kept in a closed container and counted after each session (scissors, knives, metal rulers, sharpeners, and even thumbtacks). Once this equipment is misused in group work, it can only be used under supervision. For example, if a client takes a pair of scissors out of the art therapy room, from that moment on, the use of scissors will be supervised. Since clients do not like to be supervised, there is collective pressure to obey the rules.

One art therapist said that she noticed that students coping with mental disorders may find it difficult to work on ongoing projects. She described a client who was working on the ongoing project, but as soon as something failed her, she ruined the artwork and did not want to go for art therapy anymore. Thus, these eventualities should be considered when suggesting a long-term complex project.

Most of the art therapists discussed the issue of the use of words in art therapy. Most felt that in individual art therapy sessions there is also a place for words, although not always and not in every situation, but they will occasionally try to ask clients something or comment on their artwork.

The house as symbolic representation of the self (Wyder, 2019)

Wyder (2019) investigated how the house, as a representation, can be used as a metaphor for the self in adolescent in-patient psychiatric art therapy. In this study, the art therapy sessions revolved around the single specific theme of the house to determine whether it would lend itself to express past and current painful experiences and help the adolescents reconstruct themselves. Based on the regular participation of nine adolescents (three males and six females), she found that clients' house drawings and paintings: (1) represent a means of expressing current mental states (e.g., they convey confinement, transition, and movement); (2) point to past painful experiences (e.g., broken, abandoned, porous, and burning houses); (3) allow for sensory and physical contact with art materials. Over time, through the art therapeutic process and by focusing on the house by re-building and re-defining the interior and exterior, she reported improvement in mental health through these topic-related aesthetic and inner transformations.

Responsive art therapy (Nielsen et al., 2019)

Responsive art therapy is a psychodynamic approach where the art therapist creates an in-session artwork as an interpretive relational response to the client's artwork. This interactive role changes the art therapist's position in the session to one of an active participant through the non-verbal communication of the art making response. The art therapist uses responsive art making to relate, inquire and empathize in a non-verbal dialogue, producing a unique form of communication: the clients have repeated experiences of expressing their emotions, feeling understood, and being responded to in a safe and non-threatening manner. Over time, the clients begin a mentalizing process, by thinking about the experiences that the images represent. Non-verbal expression becomes verbal and clients are better able to engage with others. In one study adolescents reported that responsive art therapy helped them learn how to express themselves safely (80%) and understand how their thoughts related to their feelings (78%) (Nielsen et al., 2019).

Group art therapy

In almost all settings, group work is also included. It allows clients to begin to connect to each other through the art materials and within a mediated and controlled environment. The art therapists described two main types of groups. The first is structured art therapy groups, in which the art therapist suggests a particular exercise to the clients to do together (e.g., each client draws a tree that represents him/her and together they build a group forest). The second type involves work in an open studio, where the art materials are presented on a kind of buffet and clients are invited to create in an "art as therapy" approach. An art therapist who has worked with inpatients who also have ASD said that she organizes some interventions in the classroom which include reflecting emotions in real time, or trying to resonate with clients to show them how others feel about their behavior.

One art therapist described a structured group that takes place in a psychiatric ward and has between two and eight participants. Each group session begins by looking at those present in the group, who was there the last time but did not come (for one reason or another) and how the group members feel at the given moment. If a new client comes in, there will be an explanation of the nature of the group, its goals, and how it will be conducted, first by the facilitators and later by clients who have been in the group for some time. To reduce anxiety, an explanation is provided about the process (the group uses art materials, no one needs to know how to draw, it is not a diagnosis, etc.). The art therapists' prime goal is that the clients not only speak to them or "through them", but learn to relate and respond to each other. To promote dialogue, they resonate and ask for reflections from the whole group about statements from each group member. During periods when the group is stable, one day a week focuses on group work and another day on individual work in a group setting. In the group work, the instruction will start with a small individual drawing that will later be placed on a joint poster board so that a joint work can be created. After deciding on the placement, and pasting the individual artworks, group members are asked to relate to the common background (the white board), create paths that connect the artworks, and decide together how they fill the joint spaces. The end of the session involves a conversation about the joint work: what it was like to create together, how someone felt when no one made a path toward him/her, who/what led the group discussions, who took the lead role and made decisions and how it felt to him/her/everyone, how those who did not take part in decisions and only followed the instructions felt, etc. During individual work in the group setting, the tasks focus on the "picture of the week". Clients are invited to depict the previous week or a significant moment by a line, blob, color, or texture. Toward the end of the session, the artworks are displayed on the wall and there is a discussion about each work (which includes a phenomenological observation and the clients' explanation of how the work was done).

Janice Shapiro, who was also interviewed for this chapter, was one of the founders of the "open studio" approach in the adolescent unit in a psychiatric hospital in Israel. She described how the unit invited all the clients to participate three times a week in the open studio, a model based on individual, non-directive artwork within a group setting, with an emphasis on the importance of the subject being chosen by the client. In addition, each client attended a weekly individual art therapy session in the same studio space. The art therapists actively reached out to all the clients to encourage them to participate. Although they were asked to be present during the whole session, this was flexible and latecomers were also welcomed. The studio offered a wide range of materials and tools to work with, from classic art materials to carpentry and welding equipment, found objects including broken ones, fabrics and threads, and more. The aim was to invite the clients to express themselves creatively and authentically. Sometimes the opening leading to realizing this aim might be through copying a picture, through working on a craft technique, or through any other activity involving tangible materials. The materials were to be found in cupboards, on shelves, in drawers, in boxes, or baskets under tables. The clients were invited to enter into a journey of exploration to search not only for their subject but also for the materials that were right for them.

This approach is in the Jungian spirit that sees the Self as the ultimate source of knowledge as to what is right for each person. In the studio, there were art books that could be used to find themes or images that feel right as a starting point (e.g., Janice described how Munch's painting "The Scream" was the subject of numerous variations throughout the years. The book about Munch literally came apart due to being used so often). At times, the clients expressed images in words and the art therapist would suggest expressing the images using materials. For example, when an adolescent told the art therapist that his life was garbage, she asked exactly what that garbage looked like and suggested he create it. When clients refused to come to the studio because they didn't like art, they were invited to come anyway and tell us what they did like. For example, someone who said he was only interested in football was invited to explain the game on paper and sketched a football field including the players. The art therapist's role was that of a "midwife", there to help give birth to a creative process, if needed. After the birth of the artwork, the therapist's interventions were mainly as a witness reflecting the value of the work as meaningful to the healing process.

A number of other art therapists who also implement the open studio approach said that art therapists or other staff members at times engage in artwork alongside the clients. The idea of integrating staff members with clients in a variety of groups is typical of several wards in the hospital and conveyed a message of the value of joint work that could serve as modeling. In one setting, the art therapist noted that the staff covered the studio's main desk with hard gray cardboard or thick brown newsprint. This served as a "holding container" for the artistic processes created on and over it. Another art therapist said that the students who come to the studio at the special school in the community where she works are either those who are particularly talented in art and love it or those who have difficulty expressing themselves verbally and the studio seems to be able to help them. Another interviewee stated that in the studio when one of the clients is dissatisfied with his/her artwork, she tells him or her to make the ugliest work possible. She then inquires whether the end result was achieved and how the student felt about it. The answer is usually that it was a lot of fun, which opens up a new space for work.

In community settings, many art therapists described projects they have done over the years with clients including an environmental sculpture or painting graffiti on a wall. In these projects, the art and the joint work are the focal points. Another art therapist who works in a closed ward in hospital brought a box with all kinds of old shoes, everyone chose a shoe and worked on it, and then these were presented in an exhibition in the ward.

Clients with eating disorders (Ben-Gal Hazan et al., 2019)

Although most of the art therapists who took part in the study described their work as dynamic and were less involved in direct interventions, about half of the therapists and roughly half of the articles saw value in having clients engage in self-image and body image work through art. The experience of creating a representation that relates to self-image in general or the body image in particular introduces the clients to one of the most difficult issues for them in treatment. The existing proof of the visual body image confronts the clients with themselves and allows for external observation. The art materials provide direct contact with the body, which makes it possible to feel where I start and where I end. This can enable clients to experience the boundaries of their body, which is not always fully clear to them. Then, the emerging image can also be processed verbally.

Art interventions can help address the restrictions that clients with eating disorders impose on themselves. Most of the art therapists who took part in the study first allowed their clients to build a safe place for themselves in the art therapy room, which provided for control and security, and later allowed other art materials to expand the options and try to release the obsession. Working with different art materials accompanies these transitions. The art and its symbolization permit clients to expand the emotional experience from "everything or nothing" to other options. Most of the art therapists raised the issue of distancing in order to talk about the other and deal indirectly with content that is difficult to express in words. According to the interviewees, their use of distancing in therapeutic sessions allows clients to enter into the metaphor and release the grip and rigidity that characterize eating disorders. The use of distancing also allows for the expression of particularly difficult emotions and release through the use of art materials.

Clients dealing with bulimia most often face difficulties with regulation. Having access to art materials in the presence of the therapist helps develop regulation and avoid extreme situations. Half of the art therapists who took part in the study used specific interventions to deal with this experience. Through art-based interventions, the therapist invites clients coping with bulimia to experience regulation and containment (e.g., working on small pages or within frames), which will later be internalized when dealing with food.

THE MEANING OF ART

The art therapists all talked about art as another way to express contents, feelings, and experiences that cannot be expressed through words. Often, through art, therapists can begin to observe what their clients are going through. One interviewee said that she believes there is something healing in connecting to creative places, places of strength and health. The content of the artwork is sometimes frightening but if the clients manage to bring that content to the art product, they are already engaged in the work and the treatment has started to occur. The ability to express feelings, to put them on paper symbolically, is what promotes change.

One art therapist commented that art opens up spaces of experience that are not constrained by the clients' self-judgments. Another therapist referred to the fact that art is the "normal" place and that contact with art materials helps clients to break free for a moment from the diagnosis and stigma. The art therapists also described clients for whom art is a tool for relaxation, even meditation. These clients seek places of tranquility and engage sometimes in slow, circular movements, sometimes jointly with the art therapist.

One of the art therapists working in a closed psychiatric ward remarked that in art therapy with clients in acute psychotic episodes there can be feelings of meaninglessness, a deep emptiness, convergence, and thoughts of death. Art reproduces strengths and allows these clients to encounter these feelings even when sinking into an inner world and experiencing a lack of control in the inner and outer world. The artistic process of clients in psychotic states deals with chaos and attempts to reorganize. Thus, the creative process within a therapeutic relationship itself requires the use of ego forces and can strengthen them.

Clients with eating disorders (Ben-Gal Hazan et al., 2019)

Most art therapists and half of the articles that took part in the study emphasized the value inherent to working with art materials, and their specific contribution to working with clients with eating disorders. Specific art materials allow for a wide range of options and flexibility. The symptom is expressed in the body but can be touched while working with the art materials, which encourages openness to further experiences. Clients can treat art materials the way they treat food. The initial contact with different materials makes it possible to deal with initial sensations of touch and feeling, which are highly connected to eating disorders.

All the art therapists and about half of the articles that took part in the study perceived art as a way to foster communication, an additional route that sometimes makes it easier to deal with direct speech. The possibility of symbolically expressing experiences and emotions through art provides a bridge to speech that is sometimes perceived as threatening. Art is a stimulus for speech and content that it is sometimes difficult to express directly.

Most of the art therapists ascribed considerable importance to encouraging clients coping with eating disorders to have fun and play with the materials. Returning to childhood allows the clients to return to pleasurable experiences. Connecting back to a place of creativity, pleasure, feeling, and touch is a significant step for these clients. The fun and play also lead to a better acquaintance with other parts of the self.

Most art therapists and roughly half of the articles that took part in the study considered that art provided a space endowed with tangible and concrete boundaries that allow clients to have an experience of control and at the same time be boundless. Clients can relax their control over the art materials, which can then spill and be messy in a protected and safe place. Art provides a varied expansive space that allows the regressive parts to be expressed in art materials while in a containing environment. The recognition of the boundaries of the page and the material leads to the beginnings of an observation of the boundaries of the self. Art liberates and gives legitimacy to the need for containment. The possibility of manifesting anger, which tends to be directed inward, underscores the power of art in expressing difficult emotions.

Most art therapists and about half of the articles that took part in the study saw art therapy as an intermediate space that allows for detachment from reality and later a connection to reality and personal content. Art also allows for emotional detachment; clients can remain in denial and implement their defense mechanisms until other pathways open up to them. At the same time, especially after a relationship of trust in the therapist has been established, some of these experiences can be connected to reality. Art allows for both self-inquiry in relation to the client's condition and comparison to the external environment; i.e., to reality. The possibility of seeing reality through art, but choosing whether to touch it and bring it into the art therapy room, is guided by the art therapist. The artworks reflect the continuum of the clients' condition during and after the therapeutic period.

Most art therapists and about half of the articles who took part in the study saw art as the third component of the client–therapist triangle, which allows for changes in distance and closeness and thus is perceived as less threatening and direct. The presence of the third component allows for development, connection, and play. Through the use of art, the experience of visibility on the paper slowly leads to an experience of visibility in life itself. The artwork is tangible, does not authorize masking and disregard, but rather confronts the defense mechanisms. The artwork becomes the focus of the interaction and serves as a mediating object. The space between the therapist, the client, and the artwork enables and facilitates direct dealing with the difficulties.

COLLABORATIVE INTERVENTIONS INVOLVING PARENTS AND STAFF MEMBERS

Working with parents

In hospital wards, contact with parents is intense. In some settings, and especially in psychiatric day hospitals, parents must take an active part in the treatment process if they want their child to be in the framework. The parents actually got into a situation where they received a psychiatric diagnosis for their child and sometimes also had to hospitalize him/her and this is always a crisis situation that elicits a wide range of emotions. Some wards have a person who works with the client him/herself and a different person who serves as a case manager and deals with parents and other external interventions. The rationale for this approach is that there should be a separation between the content that clients express in therapy and work with their parents. In other wards, the art therapist who works with clients also meets with their parents. Here, the governing idea is that the therapist can promote a better integration and better understanding of the client's full "story", thus can also serve the client better. One of the art therapists described her involvement in the client's transition from the hospital back into the community, including training the staff in the post-hospital framework. In hospitals and especially day hospitalization, parents are sometimes encouraged to engage in parent–child art psychotherapy. This can at times include the art therapist who works with the child or adolescent and the therapist who works with the parents, resulting in four participants in the art therapy room.

Art therapists working in special schools in the community for students with mental disorders mentioned different ways to stay in touch with parents. Some schools run parents' groups, where parents can meet other parents who have children with mental disorders, and share feelings and experiences. Sometimes these sessions involve art-based interventions (e.g., guided imagery when they imagine a moment of closeness with their child), where the goal is to learn how to better understand their children and how they can help them.

Working with staff members

In special schools in hospitals, the staff work is closely coordinated, especially between the art therapist working with the client and the case manager who is also a therapist. The art therapists often make it clear to clients that their confidentiality is maintained at the level of the entire staff, so that staff members can pass on information to each other. In their capacity as case managers, art therapists sometimes also help mediate between a particular teacher and a client when issues arise. Staff meetings are frequent, and there is a tight collaboration between the staff on the ward and the school staff. The goal of these staff meetings is to achieve a broader perspective on the clients in a variety of situations which can show that a client who is thriving in art therapy may have a variety of difficulties elsewhere. One art therapist emphasized that since clients use numerous defense mechanisms, they sometimes create projections and splits in the staff that are highly diagnostic and need to be taken into account. In addition, art therapists often conduct workshops for the educational and/or medical staff in order to make their tools accessible and explain their work in the art therapy room. One art therapist said that they allow staff to attend the open studio and invite them to create their emotional response to a particular client. In this way, aspects of countertransference can be better understood, and what the client evokes in various staff members.

In the special schools in the community, teamwork is closely coordinated as well. Significant in-depth work on each client is carried out and the art therapists also help teachers and assistants deal with the emotional aspects of the students who are not always their clients. The art therapists working in these schools emphasized the complexity of the ethical aspects involved where they have to choose what is appropriate to disclose from the art therapy room and what is not needed. This requires considerable understanding on the part of both the educational staff and the therapeutic staff and is not straightforward.

CLINICAL ILLUSTRATION

Lital, a skinny 13-year-old girl, came to a psychiatric inpatient ward after being severely sexually abused. Her condition deteriorated, she functioned increasingly less well and cried more often. She came to the ward like a small, injured animal who would cry, howl, lie on the floor, and barely communicate with her surroundings. After an evaluation, she was placed on medication and referred for intensive art therapy.

In the first sessions even in the art therapy room, she sprawled on the floor, whimpering and in tears. She was curled up inside herself and did not seem to notice the art therapist at all. The art therapist observed her for one session and brought finger paints to the next session and placed a small dollop of paint next to Lital. Lital continued to cry and howl but her hand began to stir the soft material and apply it slowly to the floor and wall next to it. The art therapist watched with interest. The sessions went on and each time Lital played with the paint puddled on the floor during the session.

After four sessions, the art therapist invited Lital to get up from the floor and handed her a tray with several pools of finger paint. Lital still cried occasionally, but there were also moments when she watched the colors mixing and gliding into each other intently. She spread the paint in every direction with her hands, some on the tray and some on her hands and arms. She seemed to relish the soft, cold touch of the material. There were a few moments when she looked up and two big green eyes peered at the art therapist.

Two sessions later the art therapist put plasticine on the table and the work surface. She sat down next to Lital and showed her how to use the plasticine. Lital looked at the material, smeared paints, and mixed them together. Quietly she took a small lump of clay and also began to smear it on the surface. The art therapist tried to explain the differences between the materials and what might happen to the clay, but Lital continued to work in great concentration. She applied, rolled, and created paint surfaces alongside the clay surfaces.

The next session, Lital returned to her work and saw that the clay had dried and crumbled. The art therapist was sure it would not be easy for Lital. Lital, however, very patiently collected the dried bits that had fallen off the work and put the fragments in a small box. Using a brush, she removed the remaining plasticine and cleaned the clay. In subsequent sessions, she continued to work with the clay, spreading it on surfaces and in the next session collecting the fragments, scraping it using tools, and carefully collecting them in the box.

This collection seemed to calm Lital down. She handled the clay gently, collecting bit after bit and sliding her hand over the smooth surface underneath. Lital had been now in the ward for two months and her condition was improving. There was still a long way to go, but the art therapist and other staff members started talking with her about moving on to the next framework. During the last session, the art therapist wondered how she would say goodbye to Lital. Lital, however, had an idea of her own. She took some water and added it to the mixture she had created. She gently mixed the clay crumbs with the water, until a new material began to crystallize. Finally, she placed the clay on the table and said to the art therapist – "You can give this to your next client…".

SUMMARY

This chapter outlined several key goals of art therapy for children and adolescents coping with mental disorders. The first involves improving their quality of life, their ability to integrate into society in the future in the best way possible, and in many cases also an attempt to help clients choose life. The second goal is to give them a space through art therapy where they can create and be heard, express their inner world, their fantasies, and feelings. The act in itself of forming a therapeutic alliance, which is often problematic, allows clients to feel meaningful to someone else. Special schools in the community implement a multi-stage process ranging from adaptation to school through preparation for the transition to the post-educational framework. Group work can address the loneliness of these clients and reinforce a sense of belonging. In clients with eating disorders, art therapy can assist them to live with their disorder and symptoms while expressing emotions, expanding and relaxing strictures, and finding ways to express the eating disorder and the accompanying symptoms in non-somatic ways.

The art therapists all described their personal dealings with very difficult cases, and the fear that can permeate into their personal lives. Psychotic processes often impede the formation of a therapeutic alliance, as is the case with eating disorders. These difficulties manifest as fear of getting into creative processes or being exposed in therapy. A lengthy courtship process is sometimes required to overcome this resistance. Interviewees who work in hospitals described the problems of wanting to provide a range of art making tools, including those that cut, and the need to protect the clients from themselves. In clients with eating disorders, recruitment for art therapy is impeded by rigidity, reduction, and perfectionism.

Most of the art therapists use a dynamic approach when working individually with clients. Clients are invited to engage in a personal journey. The art therapists provide the art materials and sometimes suggest specific techniques to expand their repertoire. In clients with eating disorders, art therapists sometimes suggest working directly on self-image and body image. Some clients can progress to reflective processes where they observe their experiences in the creative process in particular and in life in general. This involves distancing and observing the metaphors that arise in treatment. Sometimes, a "house" can act as a symbolic representation of the self. Art therapists also occasionally use responsive art therapy to help clients. When the work is done in a group setting, it is usually divided into two main approaches. One involves structured groups, in which the work revolves around exercises, themes, and techniques suggested by the art therapist. The second allows clients to continue working on individual art pieces in the open studio, in which case they are assisted by the art therapist in the presence of group members. Sometimes staff members are also invited to engage in artwork along with the clients.

REFERENCES

Acharya, M., Wood, M., & Robinson, P. (1995). What can the art of anorexic patients tell us about their internal world: A case study. *European Eating Disorders Review*, 3(4), 242–254.

Beck, E. H. (2007). *Art therapy with an eating disordered male population: A case study* (Master's thesis of Drexel University. Philadelphia, PA).

Ben-Gal Hazan, R., Carmon, P., Regev, D., & Snir, S. (2019). The unique contribution of art therapy in the field of eating disorders. *The Academic Journal of Creative Arts Therapies*, 9(2), 951–964. (In Hebrew).

Braito, I., Rudd, T., Buyuktaskin, D., Ahmed, M., Glancy, C., & Mulligan, A. (2021). Systematic review of effectiveness of art psychotherapy in children with mental health disorders. *Irish Journal of Medical Science* (1971-), 1–15.

Edwards, C. (2008). Bringing "The World" into the room: Art therapy, women and eating issues. In S. L. Brooke (Ed.). *The Creative Therapies and Eating Disorders* (vol. 3, pp. 28–55).

Harnden, B. (1995). *Starving for expression inside the secret theatre: An art and drama therapy group with individuals suffering from eating disorders* (Master's thesis of Concordia University Montreal. Quebec, Canada).

Jeong, H., & Kim, Y. (2006). Art therapy: Another tool for the treatment of anorexia nervosa. *Psychiatry Investigation*, 3(1), 107.

Lyshak-Stelzer, F., Singer, P., Patricia, S. J., & Chemtob, C. M. (2007). Art therapy for adolescents with posttraumatic stress disorder symptoms: A pilot study. *Art Therapy*, 24(4), 163–169.

Malchiodi, C. A. (1999). *Medical art therapy with children*. Jessica Kingsley Publishers.

Matto, H. (1997). An integrative approach to the treatment of women with eating disorders. *The Arts in Psychotherapy*, 24(4), 347–354.

Naitove, C. E. (1986). "Life's but a walking shadow": Treating anorexia nervosa and bulimia. *Arts in Psychotherapy*, 13(2), 107–119.

Nielsen, F., Isobel, S., & Starling, J. (2019). Evaluating the use of responsive art therapy in an inpatient child and adolescent mental health services unit. *Australasian Psychiatry*, 27(2), 165–170.

Schaverien, J. (1994). The transactional object: Art psychotherapy in the treatment of anorexia. *British Journal of Psychotherapy*, 11(1), 46–61.

Tyson, E. H., & Baffour, T. D. (2004). Arts-based strengths: A solution-focused intervention with adolescents in an acute-care psychiatric setting. *The Arts in Psychotherapy*, 31(4), 213–227.

Ugurlu, N., Akca, L., & Acarturk, C. (2016). An art therapy intervention for symptoms of post-traumatic stress, depression and anxiety among Syrian refugee children. *Vulnerable Children and Youth Studies*, 11(2), 89–102.

Wolf, J. M., Willmuth, M. E., & Watkins, A. (1986). Art therapy's role in the treatment of anorexia nervosa. *American Journal of Art Therapy*, 25(2), 39–46.

Wyder, S. (2019). The house as symbolic representation of the self: Drawings and paintings from an art therapy fieldwork study of a closed inpatient adolescents' focus group. *Neuropsychiatrie de l'Enfance et de l'Adolescence*, 67(5–6), 286–295.

BRIEF BIOGRAPHIES OF THE ART THERAPISTS WHO CONTRIBUTED TO THIS CHAPTER

Liela Abramovich, art therapist (M.A.), Jungian sand play therapist, supervisor, and lecturer at the Kibbutzim College, has worked for 23 years at the Geha Educational Center in the closed psychiatric ward for adolescents with mental disorders at the Geha Mental Health Center.

Pazit Carmon, art therapist (M.A.) and supervisor, is a graduate of a psychoanalytic psychotherapy program, and has worked for 20 years as an art therapist. She is specialized in the treatment and diagnosis of eating disorders at the Eating Disorders Clinic at Rambam Medical Center in Haifa.

Tal Domoshevizki-Oren, art therapist (M.A.) and supervisor, has worked for 12 years as an art therapist in special education settings for hospitalized students with Autism Spectrum Disorder (ASD) who need psychiatric treatment.

Daniela Finkel, art therapist (Ph.D. student), Jungian sand play therapist, supervisor, and lecturer at the Kibbutzim College and Bar Ilan University, has worked for 15 years with children and adolescents with mental disorders at the Merhavim Mental Health Center in Beer Yaakov – Ness Ziona.

Carmit Gal-Nes, art therapist (M.A.) and supervisor, has worked for ten years as an art therapist in special education settings for students with mental disorders.

Vardit Gvuli-Margalit, art therapist (M.A.) and supervisor, has worked for 27 years as an art therapist, including 22 years in special education setting for hospitalized students with mental disorders at the Maale Hacarmel Mental Health Center.

Rotem Ben-Gal Hazan, art therapist (M.A.), has worked for five years as an art therapist, and wrote her M.A. thesis on "The unique contribution of art therapy in the field of eating disorders".

Tehila Peleg, art therapist (M.A.) and supervisor, has worked for 13 years as an art therapist, including 7 years in special education settings for hospitalized students with mental disorders.

Janice Shapiro, art therapist (M.A.) and supervisor, Jungian analyst, lecturer at the ASA – Ono Academic College, has worked for 30 years as an art therapist with adolescents coping with mental disorders, in the adolescent unit of Eitanim Psychiatric Hospital.

Meirav Tal, art therapist (M.A.) and supervisor, has worked for 11 years in the Ziv Special Education School at the Ziv Medical Center for Child and Adolescent Mental Health.

Ofra Yarkoni, art therapist (M.A.) and supervisor, has worked for 25 years as an art therapist, including 3 years in special education settings for students with mental disorders.

Index

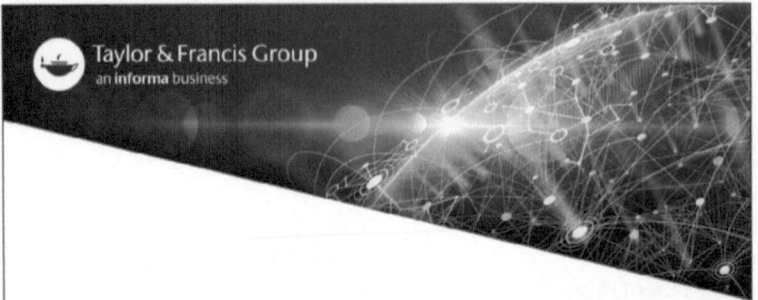
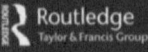
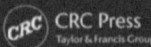